AF598062

New Techniques for Thoracic Outlet Syndromes

J. Ernesto Molina

New Techniques for Thoracic Outlet Syndromes

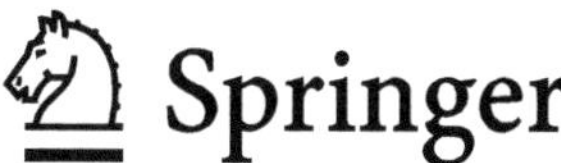

J. Ernesto Molina, MD, PhD
Division of Cardiothoracic Surgery
University of Minnesota
Minneapolis, MN, USA

ISBN 978-1-4614-5470-0 ISBN 978-1-4614-5471-7 (eBook)
DOI 10.1007/978-1-4614-5471-7
Springer New York Heidelberg Dordrecht London

Library of Congress Control Number: 2012950462

Printed on acid-free paper

Springer is part of Springer Science+Business Media (www.springer.com)

[Wir] dürfen uns nicht mit unseren Leistungen brüsten und sie als ein Ende ansehen. Eine neue Zeit wird kommen mit neuen Lehren und neuen Ideen. Sorgen wir dass wir aufnahmebereit sind und ihr Verständnis entgegenbringen.

[We may not boast with our accomplishments seeing them as a final end point. New times will come with new advances and new ideas. We should concern ourselves to be ready and to spread that knowledge.]

Ferdinand Sauerbruch
"Das war mein Leben"
Kindler Verlag Publ. München 1951

With gratitude and devotion to
God our Lord
Who granted me the time to be of service
to these patients suffering from Thoracic
Outlet Syndrome
who trusted the work of my hands.
To the inspiration and celestial light of the
Holy Virgin Mary.
To my devoted wife Carmen Aida
loyal companion throughout my entire life.
To the nurses who rendered their
unselfish service
to each and every patient entrusted
to their care.

Preface

Thoracic outlet syndromes being neurogenic-arterial, venous, or caused by the presence of a cervical rib or other anomalies affect mostly young people comprising from teenagers to middle-aged people, most of them in their productive years and fully active physically, either at work or in sports. Throughout the years, many approaches and treatments have been proposed to deal with this problem. However, most of the information regarding thoracic outlet is found only as journal articles or short chapters included in regular surgery textbooks. Currently a textbook dedicated to thoracic outlet syndromes to help physicians involved in caring for these patients does not exist. This book presents in a comprehensive format, the newest state of the art where the physicians encountering this entity can refer to in consultation to properly treat these patients using the resources that modern medicine offers. This is more relevantly shown in the chapter dedicated to the venous thoracic outlet syndrome in which the interventional radiologist and the surgeon together are the combination team that will provide 100 % cure for that problem. The book offers the newer surgical approaches that have been developed during the past 25 years. Some of the techniques described in the section dedicated to the neurogenic syndrome are modification of operations that were proposed previously but were not fully effective and left many patients suffering with permanent disability. A compendium of the proper management of these patients that cannot be found in isolated reports of literature is presented offering the most acceptable and effective methods to handle thoracic outlet syndromes.

Acknowledgments

Editing

For the editing of this book, I am indebted to my good friend from our years of training in Minnesota, brilliant colleague, and outstanding academician Dr. Wallace P. Ritchie Jr., MD, PhD, who made possible the organization and orientation of, and gave proper direction to, all this material. His stellar career includes graduating from Johns Hopkins University Medical School and post graduate education at the University of Minnesota. He is a former Professor of Surgery at the University of Virginia, Professor of Surgery and Chairman of the Department of Surgery of Temple University School of Medicine, Executive Director/Secretary Treasurer of the American Board of Surgery, Chief of Gastrointestinal Surgery at Walter Reed Army Institute of Research, invited speaker and lecturer at many institutions and meetings, and author of over 300 publications and presentations.

His outstanding guidance and judgment made this book possible.

Interventional Radiology

The work on the venous thoracic outlet syndrome (Paget–Schroetter) would not have been possible without the total support from the Interventional Radiology Division under the leadership of David W. Hunter, MD and Charles W. Dietz, MD, who provided complete commitment and cooperation, which continues to the present day, in implementing the two-team approach, i.e., Radiology–Surgery, which achieved the present outstanding results treating this disease.

Secretarial Staff

The secretarial transcription work is appreciably acknowledged and consists of Mr. Richard A. Castillo, Executive Office and Administrative Specialist, and Mrs. Debra Gutzman, who dedicated long hours to this endeavor.

To the Copyright Clearance Center service and the publishers who granted permission for reproduction of some of the illustrations that previously appeared in the following surgical journals:

- *Annals of Thoracic Surgery*
- *Journal of Vascular Surgery*
- *Seminars in Vascular Surgery*
- *International Journal of Angiology*
- *Journal of the American College of Surgeons*

Contents

Definition of the Entities

The historical aspects of the diagnosis and treatment of thoracic outlet syndromes are important for several reasons: first, they tell us how we arrived at our current level of expertise in this regard and identify the pioneers who preceded us in this effort; secondly, the information serves as a platform from which to lead us to find the proper sources and to develop new and better methods to treat these syndromes more effectively.

Three separate entities comprise the "family" called the thoracic outlet syndromes. The first is called the neurogenic-arterial thoracic outlet syndrome, which is a separate entity with different etiology and different treatment from the second condition, the venous thoracic outlet syndrome. The third, less frequently seen than the other two, is related to congenital anomalies resulting in neurogenic and arterial symptoms related to the presence of cervical ribs or to fusion of the first and second ribs. Although all three are called thoracic outlet syndromes, the term "outlet" applies only to the first and the third. The brachial plexus, which is the affected structure in the neurogenic thoracic outlet syndrome, originates in the cervical spine and from there it runs over the rib cage to reach the arm; it provides branches for not only the arm but also the chest wall muscles. However, the nerves do not come from the chest to the outside as the name outlet would signify. The only structure that exits the chest cavity and reaches the arm is the subclavian artery. In contrast, the venous thoracic outlet syndrome is actually a problem of the "inlet" to the chest where the subclavian vein enters the mediastinum running over the first rib. These entities are very different (these historical aspects will be described separately in the individual sections of this book). Failure to recognize this fact has resulted in many reports which intermix the results treating neurogenic compression with results obtained treating venous compression occurring at the upper aperture of the chest cavity. I have made an attempt to separate these entities in order to give the reader a more precise appreciation of what we call the neurogenic thoracic outlet syndrome and the clinical picture of venous compression (usually related to a Paget–Schroetter syndrome or effort thrombosis of the subclavian vein). The treatment of this last has expanded significantly to include other aspects of subclavian vein obstruction which are mostly iatrogenic entities resulting from implantation of central venous catheters and transvenous devices to treat cardiac arrhythmias (e.g., pacemaker and defibrillator leads). Implants of dialysis catheters and other type of lines used for administration of antibiotics or chemotherapeutic agents for prolonged periods of time have also introduced cases of venous obstructions, which, sadly, are difficult to treat with fewer experienced physicians able to solve them. A major purpose of this book is to help guide new surgeons to the appropriate treatment of these new complex problems. In particular, I wish to make them aware of procedures which have been found ineffective in the past.

The principal point is this: basically, two general types of acquired thoracic outlet syndromes exist, each of which requires a different therapeutic approach. The widespread lack of appreciation of the distinction between these entities is derived from the fact that much of the published literature consists of series of cases in which both types have been admixed. The end-result: patients run the risk of undergoing an inappropriate operative procedure.

As a rough guide, expanded upon below, a patient presenting in a non-emergent setting complaining of weakness and parasthesias of the arm and fingers is different from the patient who shows up in the emergency room with a severely swollen arm in pain due to obstruction of the venous return circulation. In the first case the most likely diagnosis is a neurogenic thoracic outlet syndrome. Because of the considerations outlined in the anatomy section, these neurogenic symptoms are often combined with compromised arterial circulation to the arm. This presentation should be called a neurogenic-arterial thoracic outlet syndrome. A second type of presentation of a patient with an acutely swollen and painful arm due to obstruction of the venous return from the arm represents a venous thoracic outlet syndrome, which most of the time does not cause either neurogenic symptoms or evidence of compromised arterial circulation. This is therefore a venous thoracic outlet syndrome, commonly referred to as effort thrombosis of the subclavian vein, or as noted, Paget–Schroetter syndrome (named after the two physicians who described this clinical picture in the nineteenth century).

In summary, the conditions addressed in this book are presented in the following order:

1. Neurogenic-arterial thoracic outlet syndrome.
2. Paget–Schroetter syndrome or venous thoracic outlet syndrome.
    (a) Acute stage.
    (b) Chronic state.
3. Cervical rib.
4. Venous obstructions due to implanted devices.
5. Other congenital anomalies.

Anatomy and Classification

For most surgeons the term thoracic outlet refers anatomically to the upper aperture of the chest cavity. It should be noted, however, that some anatomy books, even recent ones, refer to the upper aperture as "inlet" and name as the "outlet" the base of the chest, the greater aperture of the rib cage in its lower portion i.e., the diaphragmatic circular space [1, 2]. Following the most common clinical interpretation, we will in this textbook identify as the thoracic outlet the upper aperture of the chest in order to avoid any confusion in terminology. This upper opening is basically delineated by the course of the first rib which originates at the first thoracic vertebral body, encircles the opening, and inserts anteriorly in the sternum below the sternoclavicular joint. The space is outlined medially by the structures located centrally, namely the trachea, esophagus, and the thoracic vertebral body. In this confined hemicircular space only one structure actually leaves the chest cavity, the subclavian artery, which then pursues its course over the first rib to reach the arm. The brachial plexus originates from the cervical spine and then follows a descending course over the first rib. Two important structures actually enter the chest in the anterior portion of this space, the subclavian vein and the thoracic duct (Fig. 1). The clavicle, which occupies a position above the level of the first rib, comes down in an acute angle to insert in the sternum and contributes only partially to form the thoracic outlet.

The components of the thoracic outlet named from front to back are (Fig. 2): First at the level of the insertion of the first rib into the sternum, a strong ligament arising from the clavicle called the costoclavicular ligament. Immediately next and in front of it is the subclavius tendon, which inserts on to the inferior aspect of the clavicle and forms a strong tendon positioned in front of the costoclavicular ligament. Together these two ligaments form a very firm and sharp ridge, which together with the first rib at the bottom form an acutely angled space through which the subclavian vein runs into the chest cavity. Immediately behind the subclavian vein, the anterior scalene muscle tendon also inserts on top of the first rib, thus completing the tunnel through which the vein travels to reach the mediastinum in the thoracic cavity. This tunnel has very definite borders therefore, all of which are very strong but which cause no problems in normal individuals (e.g., obstruction to flow in the subclavian vein). The study reported by Matsumura [3] shows the dynamics of the arm movements (observed

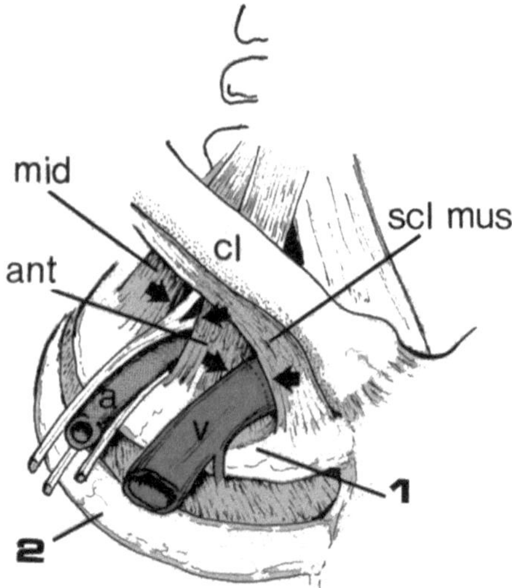

Fig. 1 Normal anatomy of the thoracic outlet on the right side. *Cl* clavicle, *Sclmus* subclavius muscle, *mid* middle scalene muscle, *ant* anterior scalene muscle. 1 = first rib, 2 = second rib, *a* = subclavian artery, *v* = subclavian vein

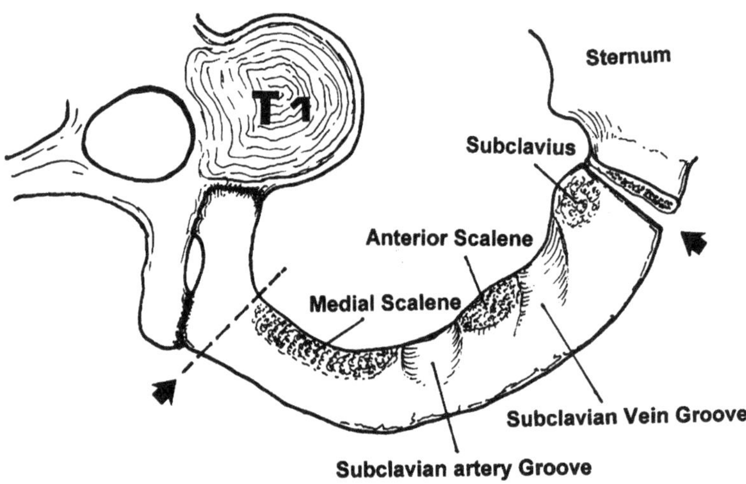

Fig. 2 Superior view of the first rib showing (*arrows*) the level at which the first rib should be divided for removal in cases with neurogenic thoracic outlet syndrome. Sites of muscle insertions are depicted

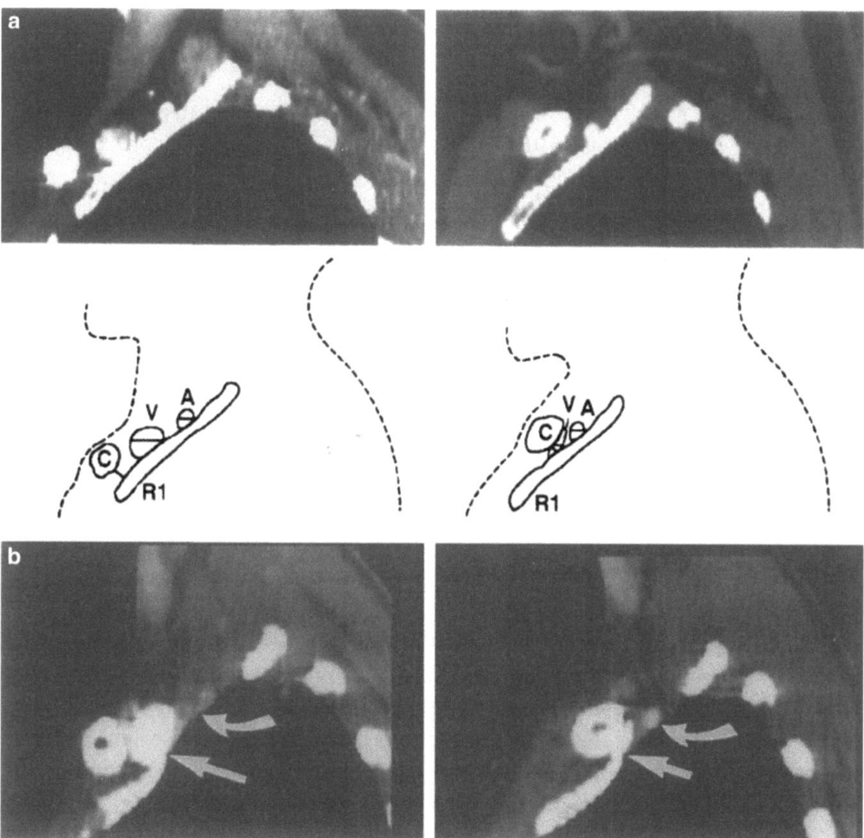

Fig. 3 Matsumura Report 1997. *Above*: Composite of sagittal CT image at costoclavicular region demonstrates neutral (*left*) and abducted positions (*right*). Posterior movement of clavicle causes scissoring impingement of the vein. Artery is posterior to swinging clavicle. *Below*: Schematic depiction of sagittal plane shows first rib (*R1*), clavicle (C), measurement of costoclavicular distance (*oblique line*), venous diameter (v), and arterial diameter (a)

using helical computer tomography) demonstrating that abduction of the arm causes posterior movement of the clavicle which results in an obvious scissoring impingement of the vein, occasionally to the point of interrupting the blood flow temporarily (Fig. 3). However in some individuals, the surrounding muscles become very prominent due either to their occupations, or to vigorous sports activities like weight lifting. Repeated movements of the arm over the head, lifting, and pushing heavy objects can lead to the thickening of both the subclavius tendon and the anterior scalene muscle tendon that contributes to a narrowing of the tunnel which over long periods of time or even acutely on occasion, especially with a sudden effort of the arms the muscles become tense and working as a vise clamp down on the vein causing injury of the endothelium leading to thrombosis (see next section on Paget–Schroetter syndrome).

Behind the anterior scalene muscle, the subclavian artery exits from the chest cavity and rides over the first rib toward the arm. Behind this artery the middle scalene

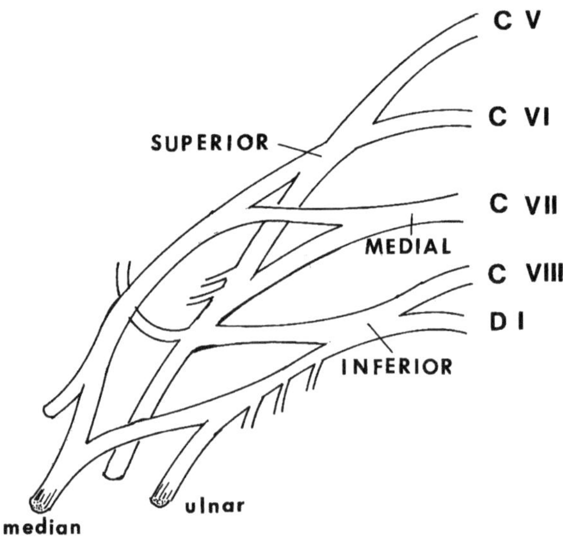

Fig. 4 Anatomical structure of the brachial plexus

muscle inserts in a long linear fashion on the upper surface of the rib extending back to the point where the first rib joins the transverse process of the T1 vertebral body (Fig. 2). The middle scalene muscle upper insertions run from C third, fourth, fifth, and sixth posterior tubercles of the transverse process. The anterior scalene inserts in the fourth, fifth, and sixth anterior tubercles of the same transverse processes. Between the fibers of the middle and the anterior scalene muscle, the nerve trunks of the brachial plexus originating at the cervical spine travel together with the subclavian artery to reach the arm. This is an area where the brachial plexus branches are intermingled with the muscle fibers and where compression of these structures can occur causing symptoms.

The structure of the brachial plexus is as follows. There are three major trunks superior, anterior, and posterior. Most of the innervation to the muscles of the forearm and hand are provided by the median and the radial nerve which run anteriorly and superiorly. The nerves innervating the ulnar area of the forearm and the third, fourth, and fifth, fingers run in the posterior trunk, which originates in the lowest portion of the cervical spine and at the level of T1 of the thoracic spine (Fig. 4).

The previous description makes clear that there are two different zones in the thoracic outlet; (Fig. 5) the anterior portion (the space through which the subclavian vein circulates) and the posterior space behind the anterior scalene muscle (through which the subclavian artery and the trunks of the brachial plexus emerge). The presence of a cervical rib or its equivalent always forces the subclavian artery into an abnormal course, riding over the cervical rib itself or its extended ligaments. This places the artery in a higher position and at a sharper angle while traveling to the arm (Fig. 6). Note: The artery never runs between the cervical rib and the first rib; it always travels over the cervical rib or its tendinous extension. In fact the space created between the cervical rib and the first rib is invariably filled with fibers belonging to the middle or the anterior scalene muscles.

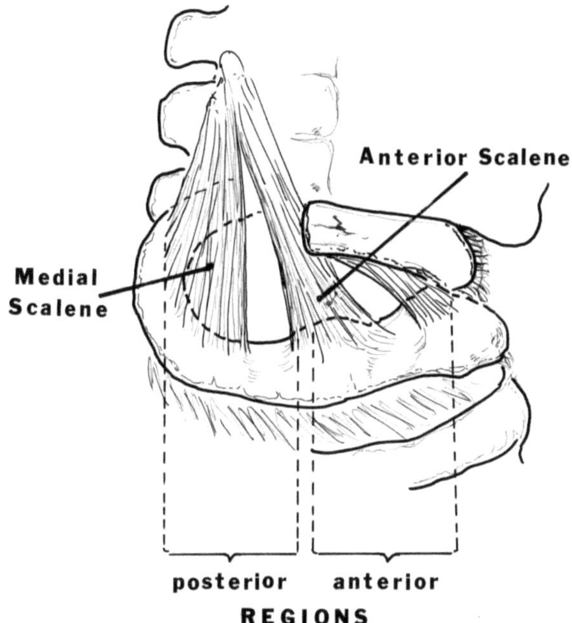

Fig. 5 This illustration shows the two regions of the thoracic outlet separated by the anterior scalene muscle. The anterior space which constitutes the inlet is outlined by the subclavius muscle the anterior scalene muscle and the first rib. The posterior space behind the anterior scalene muscle shows the separation between the anterior scalene muscle and the medial which constitutes the "trigonum costal-interscalenicum" of Puusepp through which the brachial plexus and the subclavian artery run. The medial scalene muscle forms a fan-shaped insertion on the superior aspect of the first rib

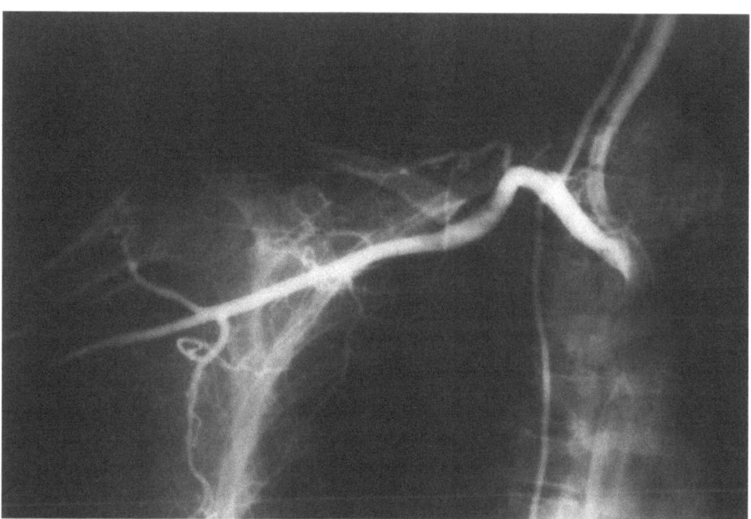

Fig. 6 Arteriogram of the right subclavian artery showing the forced superior course of the subclavian artery passing over the cervical rib before reaching the arm

According to Sanders and Roos [4, 5], the triangular space formed by the anterior and middle scalene muscles and the first rib has several differing configurations in humans. The nerve trunks that cross this space arise at different levels. In cadavers of both genders the nerves emerged higher in the triangle in those who had had symptoms of the neurogenic thoracic outlet syndrome than in those who were asymptomatic. (The differences were greater in women than in men). It is probable that, when the muscles contract, they exert a pinching mechanism on the nerve trunks that may on occasion involve the subclavian artery. The age-related sagging of the shoulder position in adults may also stretch the scalene muscles to a more acute angle at the level where the nerve trunks emerge. This may explain why in childhood or even in puberty, the patients may not have symptoms but until later in adulthood particularly in women who experience a greater shoulder descent to a more sloping position, as suggested by Naffziger and Grant [6] in their excellent monograph. Loss of muscular tone and drooping of the shoulders with aging may have the same effect regardless of gender.

Compression of the brachial plexus trunks constitutes what we call a neurogenic thoracic outlet syndrome. In 51 % of the cases it involves compression of the subclavian artery as well [7–9]. Both structures are affected because of their common position in the posterior triangular space of the thoracic outlet.

Another important anatomic consideration is the position of the phrenic nerve. In the neck the nerve crosses diagonally in front of the anterior scalene muscle as it reaches the first rib. At the level of the clavicle the nerve usually separates from the anterior scalene muscle to enter the mediastinum behind the first rib. Therefore in the infraclavicular portion of the scalene muscle the phrenic nerve is already away from the muscle tendon and becomes medial following the course of the superior vena cava. This has surgical implications on the approach to be implemented when operative interventions are aimed to relieve compression of the thoracic outlet.

References

1. Kelley LL, Petersen CM. Sectional anatomy for imaging professionals. 2nd ed. St. Louis: Mosby/Elsevier; 2007. p. 276–8.
2. Mackinnon S, Patterson GA, Urschel Jr. HC. Thoracic outlet syndromes (Chapter 52). In: Thoracic surgery. 2nd ed. New York: Churchill Livingston Publishers; 2002. p. 1393–1415.
3. Matsumura JS, Rilling WS, Pearce WH, Nemecek AA, Vogelzang RL, Yao JST. Helical computed Tomography of the normal thoracic outlet. J Vasc Surg. 1997;26:776–83.
4. Sanders RJ, Roos DB. The surgical anatomy of the scalene triangle. Contemp Surg. 1989;35:11–16.
5. Roos DB. The place for scalenectomy and first-rib resection in thoracic outlet syndrome. Surgery. 1982;92:1077–85.
6. Naffziger HC, Grant WT. Neuritis of the brachial plexus mechanical in origin: the scalenus syndrome. Surg Gynecol Obstet. 1938:67;722–30.
7. Rosati LM, Lord JW. Neurovascular compression syndromes of the shoulder girdle. Modern surgical monographs. New York: Grune & Stratton; 1961. p. 168–76.
8. Molina JE, D'Cunha J. The vascular component in neurogenic-arterial thoracic outlet syndrome. Int J Angiol. 2008;17:83–7.
9. Eklof B. Vascular compression syndromes of the upper extremity. Acta Chir Scand. 1976;142:74–7.

Part I
Neurogenic-Arterial Thoracic Outlet Syndrome

Chapter 1
Symptoms of Neurogenic-Arterial Thoracic Outlet Syndrome

Commonly the symptoms associated with neurogenic compression are pain, paresthesias, numbness, tingling, and, occasionally, weakness of the hand muscles of the involved arm. Less frequently, associated arterial compression may produce paleness of the arm particularly when it is elevated to 90° or 180° of abduction [1–11]. These symptoms may be present for months or sometimes even years without producing any complications. As the symptoms progress, however, the entire hand and sometimes part of the forearm may become involved. Over 85% of patients with advanced disease complain of pain, numbness, and tingling of the hand and fingers [8, 9, 12–14]. All of them, however, will complain of a throbbing type of pain involving the entire arm, including the forearm and the hand, when the arm is abducted 90° to the shoulder level, or above that level (i.e., when they try to reach over their heads). Many times the patients cannot raise the arm over their head because of the tightening and pain experienced not only around the forearm but also around the shoulder, extending on occasion to the back at the base of the neck. As the symptoms become more severe patients may have difficulty driving their vehicles because they are unable to maintain their arms on the steering wheel preferring to keep them in their laps. Discomfort of this severity is present in 100% of cases and causes most patients to seek medical attention. The patients who suffer concomitantly from subclavian artery compression demonstrate immediate paleness of the hand upon elevation of the arm over their heads which rapidly returns to normal as it is lowered.

Because the diagnosis of neurogenic compression alone is strictly clinical, the physician must pay very careful attention to all of the symptoms of which patient complains of before examining the patient, or ordering any laboratory tests. Some have already been subjected to carpal tunnel surgery in the past due to misdiagnosis, needless to say that the symptoms do not resolve after such surgical procedures. It is important to note in this regard that the compression of the brachial plexus at the thoracic outlet affects mostly the fourth and fifth fingers of the hand whereas the carpal tunnel syndrome affects most commonly the distribution of the radial nerve (the thumb, the index and middle fingers) (Fig. 1.1). In severe cases patients learn to restrict the use of the affected arm so that even simple tasks as typing or writing

J.E. Molina, *New Techniques for Thoracic Outlet Syndromes*,
DOI 10.1007/978-1-4614-5471-7_1, © Springer Science+Business Media New York 2013

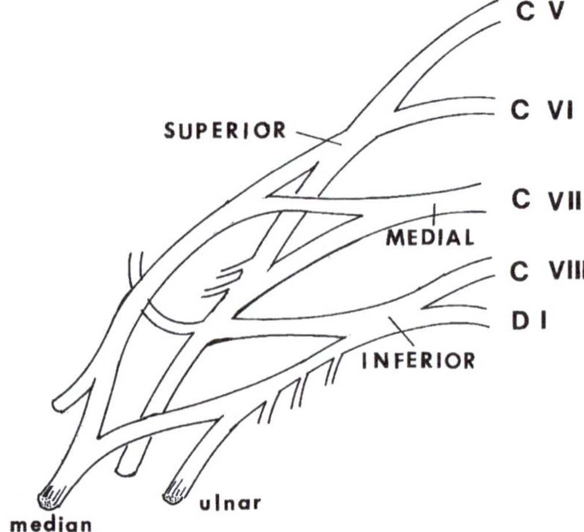

Fig. 1.1 Anatomical structure of the brachial plexus

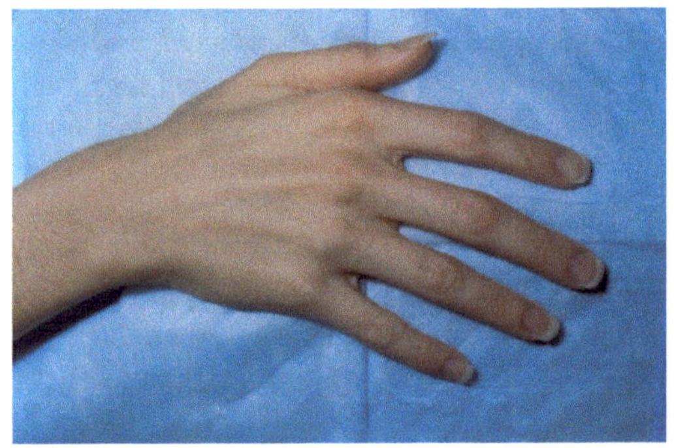

Fig. 1.2 31-year-old woman showing already atrophy of the interosseous muscles caused by the presence of cervical rib and long-standing neurogenic thoracic outlet syndrome symptoms

at a desk, or even reading a newspaper become increasingly difficult. A common complaint in women is that they are unable to comb their hair or hold a hair dryer at the level of their heads. Weakness of the hand muscles is observed in approximately 8 or 9% cases leading to lack of dexterity (e.g., dropping objects held in their hands). In far advanced cases severe damage to the nerve trunks leads to muscle atrophy and inability to use the extremity at all (Figs. 1.2 and 1.3). We have seen this in only about 2% of patients probably because they seek medical attention early when the symptoms are constant and severe preventing atrophy to occur.

In a very few cases, aneurysm of the subclavian artery may develop when the artery is compromised. Fortunately, this complication is rarely seen today because patients seek medical attention earlier than in the past. In our experience in over 200 cases operated with this syndrome we have encountered only one instance in which the patient developed an aneurysm with thrombosis of the subclavian artery and peripheral embolism to the fingers and the hand with early gangrene. The precise cause of other more rare symptoms that we have seen associated with the syndrome is more difficult to define clearly due to brachial plexus compression: In two

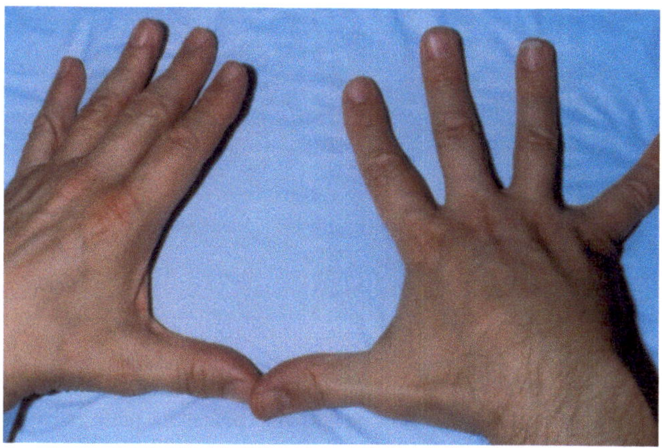

Fig. 1.3 Hands of a 46-year-old man showing atrophy of the thenar muscles on the left side. This patient has also chronic severe symptoms of neurogenic thoracic outlet syndrome

instances we have seen young women who had developed migraine headaches accompanied by nausea, and vomiting triggered by elevation of the arm over their head. In one of these cases a young school teacher had to leave her profession because she was unable to raise the arm high enough to write on the classroom blackboard. Every time she did so, she developed acute dizziness, migraine, and vomiting. These episodes lasted for 3 or 4 h even after bringing the arm back down to its normal position, and assuming a prone position. The nausea in particular persisted until about 3 or 4 h had passed. CT scans and MRIs of the brain were negative. However a very thorough examination and history strongly suggested the presence of a thoracic outlet syndrome. After operation, her symptoms disappeared and she went back to her occupation without restrictions.

The neurogenic-arterial thoracic outlet syndrome as explained above is characterized by compression of the brachial plexus trunks and most commonly the posterior trunk which is the most inferior in the bundle. From the anatomical description provided in the previous section, it is easy to understand that nerve compression may be associated with arterial compression as well [15–18], because both of these structures travel in the interscalene triangle. Although multiple publications have been written describing the association of these symptoms most of the reports were based on subjective clinical interpretation of physical maneuvers. It was not until 2008 that an objective standard duplex ultrasound test (Fig. 1.4a, b) was utilized to assess the association of arterial compression with the neurogenic component [19]. In this study it was found that 51% of the patients having neurogenic compression indeed had clear objective signs of arterial compression. If this study is positive, it is usually not necessary to proceed to CT scanning (Fig. 1.5), MRI, or more invasive tests of arteriography (Fig. 1.6a, b). On the other hand when the ultrasound test is negative there is no currently known objective radiological or laboratory based test to tell us whether or not an isolated nerve compression at the thoracic compression outlet level exists. The

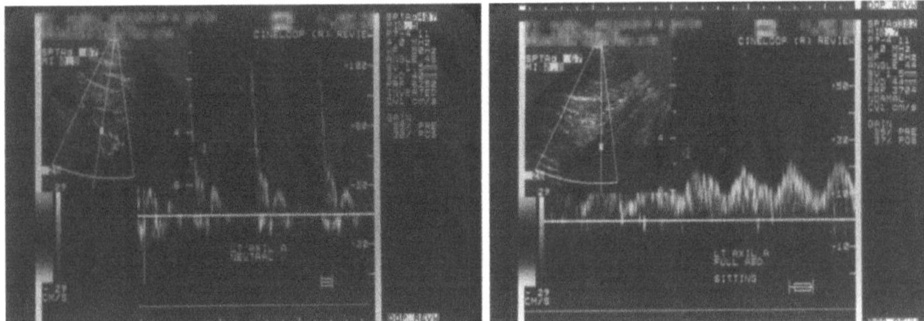

Fig. 1.4 22-year-old man with symptoms of neurogenic arterial thoracic outlet syndrome. (**a**) Arterial tracing with the arm in the neutral position. (**b**) The same patient showing the arterial tracings with the arm in full abduction showing the dampening of the pulse and tripling increase in the velocity

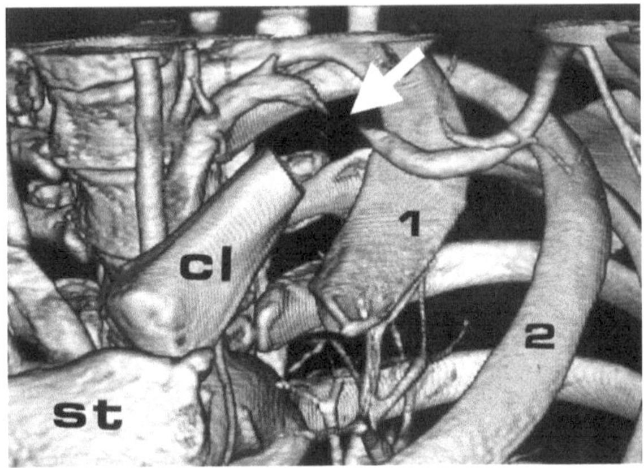

Fig. 1.5 A CT angiogram of a 26-year-old man with the left arm in full abduction showing (*arrow*) severe obstruction of the subclavian artery. Cl=clavicle (the distal end of the clavicle had been subtracted by radiologic techniques). St=sternum, 1=first rib, 2=second rib

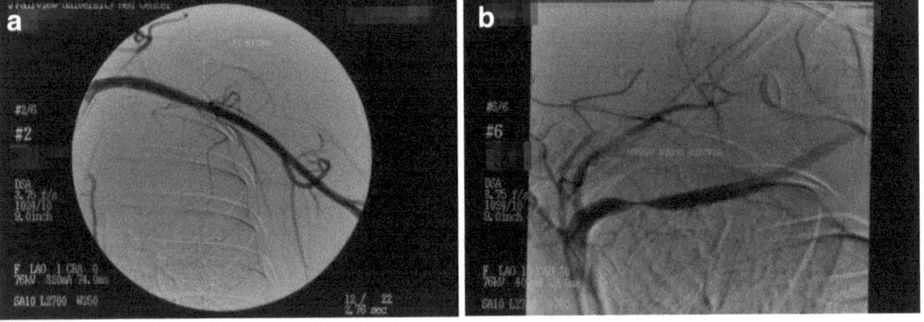

Fig. 1.6 (**a**) Arteriogram obtained in an 18-year-old woman with the arm in the normal neutral position. (**b**) The same patient with the arm in 90° abduction showing the severe pinching of the subclavian artery at the thoracic outlet

diagnosis must be made clinically. In the presence of an abnormal cervical rib, the triangle between the scalene muscles is even more severely narrowed and therefore more likely to compress the nerve trunks and artery. Even though the presence of a cervical rib is congenital, many individuals grow into adulthood without having any complaints related to it until they are in their 30s or even 40s. It is common also for a child with a cervical rib to start having symptoms at an early age, particularly if actively engaged in sports. Some do not complain of pain or discomfort until they have become fully active as teenagers. It should also be noted that patients with neurogenic-arterial thoracic outlet syndrome very rarely have an associated venous obstructive component.

In conclusion the neurogenic-arterial thoracic outlet syndrome occurs when the nerve roots with or without arterial participation are compressed in the posterior interscalenic triangle with or without the presence of cervical rib. The typical symptoms with which the patient presents may occasionally be associated with a wide variety of other complaints as noted in this chapter.

References

1. Leffert RD. Thoracic outlet syndromes. Hand Clin. 1992;8:285–97.
2. Bertelsen S. Neurovascular compression syndromes of the neck and shoulder. Acta Chir Scand. 1969;135:137–48.
3. Mackinnon S, Patterson GA, Urschel Jr HC. Chapter 52: Thoracic outlet syndromes. In: Thoracic surgery. 2nd ed. New York: Churchill Livingston; 2002. p. 1393–415.
4. Capistrant TD. Thoracic outlet syndrome cervical strain injury. Minn Med. 1986;69:13–7.
5. Telford ED, Mottershead S. The “Costoclavicular Syndrome”. Br Med J. 1947;15:325–8.
6. Griffth Pearson F. Chapter 50: Thoracic outlet syndrome. In: Mackinnon S, Patterson GA, editors. Thoracic surgery. New York: Churchill Livingston; 1995. p. 1294–8.
7. Urschel Jr HC, Razzuk MA. Chapter 18: Thoracic outlet syndrome. In: Sabiston DC, Spencer F, editors. Surgery of the chest. 5 (7 and 8)th ed. Philadelphia: Saunders; 1990. p. 536–53.
8. Rosati LM, Lord JW. Neurovascular compression syndromes of the shoulder girdle, Modern surgical monograph. New York: Grune & Stratton Inc; 1961. pp 168.
9. Altobelli GG, Kudo T, Haas BT, Chandra FA, Moy JL, Ahn SS. Thoracic outlet syndrome: pattern of clinical success after operative decompression. J Vasc Surg. 2005;42:122–8.
10. Keen WW. The symptomatology, diagnosis and surgical treatment of cervical ribs. Am J Med Sci. 1907;133(2):173–218.
11. Murphy T. Brachial neuritis caused by pressure of first rib. Aust Med J. 1910;25:582–6.
12. Molina JE. Combined posterior and transaxillary approach for neurogenic thoracic outlet syndrome. J Am Coll Surg. 1998;187:39–45.
13. Morley J. Brachial plexus neuritis due to a normal first thoracic rib: its diagnosis and treatment by excision of rib. Clin J. 1913;42:461–8.
14. Urschel Jr HC, Paulson DL, McNamara JJ. Thoracic outlet syndrome. Ann Thorac Surg. 1968;6:1–10.
15. Eastcott HHG. Cervical rib and thoracic outlet compression and other causes of upper limb occlusion. In: Arterial surgery. London: Pitman Med Publ; 1971. p. 216–34.

16. Urschel Jr HC. Chapter 19: Thoracic outlet syndromes. In: Kaiser LR, Kron IL, Spray FL, editors. Mastery of cardiothoracic surgery. Philadelphia: Lippincott-Raven; 1998. p. 178–85.
17. Ferguson TB, Burford TH, Roper CL. Neurovascular compression at the superior thoracic aperture. Surgical management. Ann Surg. 1968;167:573–9.
18. Loh CS, Wu AV, Stevenson IM. Surgical decompression for thoracic outlet syndrome. J R Coll Surg Edinb. 1989;34:66–8.
19. Molina JE, D'Cunha J. The vascular component in neurogenic-arterial thoracic outlet syndrome. Int J Angiol. 2008;17:83–7.

Chapter 2
The Diagnostic Tests

Duplex Ultrasound

As mentioned in the previous section, not every case of neurogenic thoracic outlet syndrome shows signs of arterial compression. In a recent study [1] 148 patients were evaluated with duplex ultrasound; when the patients were subjected to routine maneuvers of abduction of the arm to elicit compression of the artery, 51% of them showed definite arterial compression, while the remaining 49% did not. Thus, the duplex ultrasound exam done as outlined by Longley et al. [2, 3] is a noninvasive reliable and reproducible test to determine if arterial compression exists. It is an objective test with clear identifiable endpoints which can be accurately reproduced. MRI, CT scan, arteriogram, or EMG tests should not be requested routinely. Clinical evaluation and duplex ultrasound are sufficient to establish the diagnosis.

Abduction Maneuvers

Most reports in the literature [4] have referred to the diagnostic value of finding a loss of pulse during several maneuvers including the Adson test, the Wright test, and simple abduction of the arm to 90° and 180° but this is a highly subjective interpretation test depending on the experience of the examiner. Often enough, however, when the radial pulse does not disappear the patients are told that they do not have thoracic outlet syndrome, and are left in an undiagnosed limbo. Among the provocative tests available to elicit the symptoms [4–7] we have found the two most important to be first the Wright maneuver in which the arm is placed in 90° abduction rotating the hand outwards. The patient turns his/her head in the opposite direction and takes a deep breath, holding on to the inspiration, all the while the radial pulse is monitored. The Adson maneuver, with abduction of the arm to 180°, may elicit the symptoms immediately. One other maneuver that may be helpful and aimed to relieve the nerve compression is asking the patient to shrug his or her shoulders up.

J.E. Molina, *New Techniques for Thoracic Outlet Syndromes*,

DOI 10.1007/978-1-4614-5471-7_2,

When the shoulder is elevated the symptoms usually go away or the patient feels better. Some of these patients have adopted the posture of having the shoulders always shrugged up above the normal level to obtain some relief of their symptoms. When these maneuvers are implemented even when the radial pulse persists, signs of neurogenic compression should be interpreted as positive.

EMG

Urschel et al. [8, 9] had reported that using electromyography to determine the velocity of nerve impulse transmission from the neck to the hand and fingers is an accurate objective test to determine the presence of neurogenic compression. These conclusions have not been verified by many later reports and by our own clinical experience [10–14]. We found that only about 2% of patients show some abnormality in the EMG results even when they had clear clinical signs of neurogenic thoracic outlet syndrome. Therefore the use of EMG is not an accurate diagnostic test in this condition, at least until the patient has developed degenerative changes in the nerve trunks and/or in the muscles innervated by them. As Leffert has stated [15], the diagnosis of neurogenic compression in the thoracic outlet syndrome remains essentially a clinical one. Several useful maneuvers have been found to be helpful. In particular, as noted, the duplex ultrasound exam is helpful in determining the need for surgical decompression of the thoracic outlet in these patients. Figure 1.6a, b, shows the typical signs of positive duplex ultrasound tracings when arterial compression exists while applying the maneuvers of abduction to the arm involved. However in the patients who have a negative duplex ultrasound exam, whether or not neurogenic compression is the correct diagnosis can only be determined clinically.

Other Tests

As noted previously the symptoms of the neurogenic thoracic outlet syndrome which, also as noted, are associated with arterial vascular compromise 50% or more of the time are caused by the compression of the brachial plexus trunks and the subclavian artery in the posterior zone of the thoracic outlet, specifically between the anterior and the medial scalene muscle. This zone is called the "trigonum costo-interscalenicum" [16, 17] which is formed by those two muscles and the floor by the first rib. To accomplish complete decompression of these structures it is necessary to remove the first rib at that level along with dividing the scalene muscles inserting onto it [18–21]. Arteriography is rarely needed and is indicated only in cases where the duplex-ultrasound shows intrinsic abnormalities of the artery like aneurysm formation or stenosis. Ct scan exam falls in this category as well. Examples of these tests are shown in Figs. 1.5 and 1.6.

References

1. Molina JE, D'Cunha J. The vascular component in neurogenic-arterial thoracic outlet syndrome. Int J Angiol. 2008;17:83–7.
2. Longley DG, Yedlicka JW, Molina JE, et al. Color Doppler ultrasound of thoracic outlet syndrome. Semin Interv Radiol. 1990;7:230–5.
3. Longley DG, Yedlicka JW, Molina JE, et al. Thoracic outlet syndrome: evaluation of the subclavian vessels by color duplex sonography. AJR Am J Roentgenol. 1992;158:623–40.
4. Bertelsen S. Neurovascular compression syndromes of the neck and shoulder. Acta Chir Scand. 1969;135:137–48.
5. Warrens AN, Heaton JM. Thoracic outlet compression syndrome: the lack of reliability of its clinical assessment. Ann Roy Coll Surg Engl. 1987;69:203–4.
6. Eklof B. Vascular compression syndromes of the upper extremity. Acta Chir Scand. 1976;142:74–7.
7. Adson AW, Coffey JR. Cervical rib. A method of anterior approach for relief of symptoms by division of the scalenus anticus. Ann Surg. 1927;85:839–57.
8. Mackinnon S, Patterson GA, Urschel Jr, HC. Ch 52: Thoracic outlet syndromes. In: F. Griffith Pearson, editor. Thoracic surgery. 2nd ed. New York: Churchill Livingston Publishers; 2002. p. 1393–415.
9. Urschel Jr HC, Razzuk MA, Wood RE, et al. Objective diagnosis (ulnar nerve conduction velocity) and current therapy of the thoracic outlet syndrome. Ann Thorac Surg. 1971;12:608–20.
10. Capistrant TD. Thoracic outlet syndrome cervical strain injury. Minn Med. 1986;69:13–7.
11. Molina JE. Combined posterior and transaxillary approach for neurogenic thoracic outlet syndrome. J Am Coll Surg. 1998;187:39–45.
12. Wood VE, Twito R, Verska JM. Thoracic outlet syndrome. The results of first rib resection in 100 patients. Orthop Clin North Am. 1988;19:131–46.
13. Sander RJ, Pearse WH. The treatment of thoracic outlet syndrome: a comparison of different operations. J Vasc Surg. 1989;10:626–34.
14. Roos DB. The place for scalenectomy and first-rib resection in thoracic outlet syndrome. Surgery. 1982;92:1077–85.
15. Leffert RD. Thoracic outlet syndromes. Hand Clin. 1992;8:285–97.
16. Puusepp L. Kompression des Plexus brachialis durch die normale Erste Brustrippe. Folia Neuropath Eston. 1931;11:93–100.
17. Gaupp E. Über die Bewegungen des menschlichen Schultergürtels und die Ätiologie der Sogennante Narkosenlähmungen Zentralblatt. Chirurgie. 1894;34:793–809.
18. Roos DB. Experience with first rib resection for thoracic outlet syndrome. Ann Surg. 1971;173:429–42.
19. Brickner WM. Brachial plexus pressure by the normal 1st rib. Ann Surg. 1927;85:858–72.
20. Stopford JSB, Telford ED. Compression of the lower trunk of the brachial plexus by a first dorsal rib with a note on the surgical treatment. Br J Surg. 1919;7:168–77.
21. Hempel GK, Rusher AH, Wheeler CJ, et al. Supraclavicular resection of the 1st rib for thoracic outlet syndrome. Am J Surg. 1981;141:213–5.

Chapter 3
Physiotherapy

In the nonoperative treatment of neurogenic thoracic outlet syndrome physiotherapy alone may help by having the patient adopt a different posture aimed at correcting the sagging of the shoulder girdle, straightening the dorsal spine and applying exercises aimed to lift the position of the first rib from an acute downwards angle to a more horizontal one. Some of these exercises are typically shown by the routine schedule proposed by the Mayo Clinic group [1]. Unfortunately, long-term results have not proven very satisfactory. In the long run symptoms persist and the patients invariably have recurrent problems for which surgery is usually the only remedy.

Treatment and Results

Shoulder-girdle exercises for thoracic-outlet syndrome: Do only those exercises marked by the instructor. At the beginning, each exercise is done ten times in succession twice a day. As the shoulders and neck gain strength, the number of times each exercise is done consecutively can be increased.

Exercises

1. Stand erect with the arms at the sides holding in each hand a 2 pound weight (sandbags, or bottles, jars, or sacks filled with sand).

   (a) Shrug the shoulders forward and upward.
   (b) Relax.
   (c) Shrug the shoulders backward and upward.
   (d) Relax.
   (e) Shrug the shoulders upward.
   (f) Relax and repeat.

J.E. Molina, *New Techniques for Thoracic Outlet Syndromes*,
DOI 10.1007/978-1-4614-5471-7_3, © Springer Science+Business Media New York 2013

2. Stand erect with the arms out straight from the sides at shoulder level; hold a 2 pound weight in each hand (palms should be down).
   (a) Raise the arms sideways and up until the backs of the hands meet above the head (keep elbows straight).
   (b) Relax and repeat. *Note*: As strength improves and exercises 1 and 2 become easier, then the weights should be made heavier, increasing to 5–10 pounds.
3. Stand facing a corner of the room with one hand on each wall, arms at shoulder level, palms forward, elbows bent, and abdominal muscles contracted.
   (a) Slowly let the upper part of the trunk lean forward and press the chest into the corner. Inhale as the body leans forward.
   (b) Return to the original position by pushing out with the hands. Exhale with this movement.
4. Stand erect with the arms at the sides.
   (a) Bend the neck to the left attempting to touch the left ear to the left shoulder without shrugging the shoulder.
   (b) Bend the neck to the right attempting to touch the right ear to the right shoulder without shrugging the shoulder.
   (c) Relax and repeat.
5. Lie face down with the hands clasped behind the back.
   (a) Raise the head and chest from the floor as high as possible while pulling the shoulders backward and the chin in. Hold this position for a count of three. Inhale as the chest is raised.
   (b) Exhale and return to the original position.
   (c) Repeat.
6. Lie down on the back with arms at the sides with a rolled towel or a small pillow under the upper part of the back between the shoulder blades and no pillow under the head.
   (a) Inhale slowly and raise the arms upward and backward overhead.
   (b) Exhale and lower the arms to the sides.
   (c) Repeat 5–20 times.

Reference

1. Peet RM, Henriksen JD, Anderson TP, Martin GM. Thoracic outlet syndrome: evaluation of the therapeutic exercise program. Proc staff Meet Mayo Clin. 1956;31:281–5.

Chapter 4
Surgical Treatment

Historical Aspects

In the second half of the nineteenth century, the combined symptoms of numbness, pain, or complete paralysis of the arm were noted. This combination was known in the German literature as "Schlafdrucklähmung" (sleep pressure paralysis) of the arm and was also known as angiospastic neuralgia [1, 2]. In 1903, Bramwell [3] clearly expressed his opinion that compression of the brachial plexus was the cause of this problem occurring between the anterior, the middle scalene muscles, and the first rib [4–7]. This space in the thoracic outlet was clearly described and named by Puusepp (or Poussep) as "trigonum costo-interscalenicum" which he identified as definitely the site of the compression of the brachial plexus. He also suggested that all symptoms could be exacerbated if the muscles were hypertrophic [2]. We have to keep in mind that the X-rays were not available until 1895; and all prior years these assumptions were based on cadaveric dissections and the clinical impression that brachial plexus compression was the cause of these symptoms. Murphy [8] in England was the first surgeon who removed a normal first rib to treat this syndrome. The patient experienced full relief of the compressive symptoms. Some [9, 10] believed that the compression was occurring between the first rib and the clavicle, causing the numbness and paralysis of the arm (narkoselähmungen). Following the publication of Bramwell's description many investigators expressed agreement with this concept [11–15]. All concurring on the need to resect the first rib to relieve compression. New thinking [14, 16] promoted the concept that sinking of the shoulder girdle caused stretching of the scalene muscles which would narrow the triangle producing compressing of the brachial plexus. In 1913 [17] it was proposed that the compression occurred at the narrow slit between the anterior and the middle scalene muscles through which the plexus passes. Many surgeons routinely resected the first rib to relieve the compression on the strength of these conclusions. Brickner [18, 19], for example, reported that he had resected the first rib in five patients with typical symptoms; optimal results were obtained in four. The operative technique used by these surgeons invariably involved a supraclavicular approach to give access to the anterior and medial scalene muscles

DOI 10.1007/978-1-4614-5471-7_4,

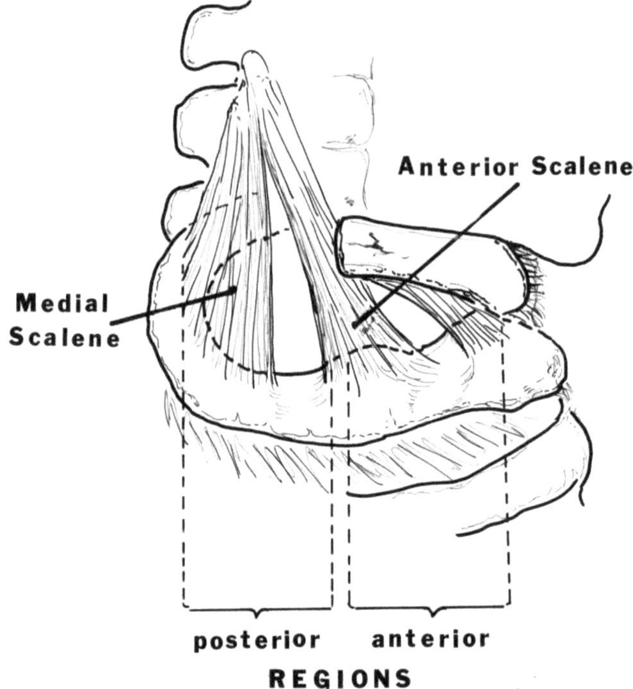

Fig. 4.1 This illustration shows the two regions of the thoracic outlet separated by the anterior scalene muscle. The anterior space which constitutes the inlet is outlined by the subclavius muscle, the anterior scalene muscle, and the first rib. The posterior space behind the anterior scalene muscle shows the separation between the anterior scalene muscle and the medial which constitutes the "trigonum costal-interscalenicum" of Puusepp through which the brachial plexus and the subclavian artery run. The medial scalene muscle forms a fan-shaped insertion on the superior aspect of the first rib

and also to the brachial plexus. Although the most anterior portion of the rib could not be removed, this was not a relevant consideration because the compression of the brachial plexus was in the posterior portion of the thoracic outlet (Fig. 4.1).

Operations aimed to remove the first rib and to divide or resect the scalene muscles involved, all originally performed using a supraclavicular approach [8, 13–15, 18, 20, 21]. This approach will be discussed later but in essence an incision is made at the anterior base of the neck allowing exposure of the scalene muscles as well as the posterior two-thirds of the first rib. The results published by these earlier investigators were "highly satisfactory" and therefore this became the recommended route to accomplish the objectives of the intervention. This approach has subsequently been promoted by many knowledgeable and competent surgeons like Stoney [13], Naffziger [14], Murphy [11], Jones [22], and many others. It has been an effective approach specifically for the neurogenic and arterial type of thoracic outlet syndrome.

References

1. Wartenberg R. Brachialgia statica paraesthetica eine Form von Akroparästhesien Journal. Z Gesamte Neurol Psychiatr. 1936;154:695–723.
2. Puusepp L. Kompression der Plexus brachialis durch die normale Erste Brustrippe. Folia Neuropath Eston. 1931;11:93–100.
3. Bramwell E. Compression of the brachial plexus between the scalene muscle and first rib. Review Neur Psych. 1903;1:236–8.
4. Roos DB. The place for scalenectomy and first-rib resection in thoracic outlet syndrome. Surgery. 1982;92:1077–85.
5. Kim D, Midha R, Murovic JA, Spinner RJ. Ch 12 subtitle, Brachial plexus anatomy and preoperative physiology. In: Kline, Hudsons, editors. Nerve injuries. 2nd ed. Philadelphia: Saunders; 2008. p. 279 (Ch 18 Thoracic Outlet Syndrome pp 373)
6. Wheeler WI de C. Compression neuritis due to the normal first dorsal rib. Practitioner. 1920;104(civ):409–18.
7. Jones FW. Variations of the first rib associated with changes in the constitution of the brachial plexus. J Anat. 1911;45:249–55.
8. Murphy JB. The clinical significance of cervical ribs. Surg Gynecol Obstet. 1906;3:514–20.
9. Gaupp E. Über die Bewegungen des menschlichen Schultergürtels und die Ätiologie der Sogennante Narkosenlähmungen Zentralblatt. Chirurgie. 1894;34:793–809.
10. Borchardt M. Symptomatologie und Therapie der Halsrippen. Berl Klin Wochenschr. 1901;38:1265.
11. Murphy T. Brachial neuritis caused by pressure of first rib. Aust Med J. 1910;25:582–6.
12. Cikrit DF, Haefner R, Nichols WK, Silver D. Transaxillary or supraclavicular decompression for the thoracic outlet syndrome: a comparison of the risks and benefits. Am Surg. 1989;55:347–52.
13. Quarfordt PG, Ehrenfeld WK, Stoney RJ. Supraclavicular radical scalenectomy and transaxillary first rib resection for thoracic outlet syndrome. A combined approach. Am J Surg. 1984;148:111–6.
14. Naffziger HC, Grant WT. Neuritis of the brachial plexus mechanical in origin. The scalenus syndrome. Surg Gynecol Obstet. 1938;67:722–30.
15. Telford ED, Mottershead S. Pressure at the cervicobrachial junction. J Bone Joint Surg Br. 1948;30:249.
16. Clagett OT. Research and prosearch. Presidential Address. J Thorac Cardiovasc Surg. 1962;44:153–66.
17. Morley J. Brachial plexus neuritis due to a normal first thoracic rib: its diagnosis and treatment by excision of rib. Clin J. 1913;42:461–8.
18. Brickner WM. Brachial plexus pressure by the normal 1st rib. Ann Surg. 1927;85:858–72.
19. Brickner WM, Milch H. First dorsal simulating cervical rib—by maldevelopment or by pressure symptoms. Surg Gynecol Obstet. 1925;40:38–44.
20. Adson AW, Coffey JR. Cervical rib. A method of anterior approach for relief of symptoms by division of the scalenus anticus. Ann Surg. 1927;85:839–57.
21. Falconer MA, Li FWP. Resection of the first rib in costoclavicular compression of the brachial plexus. Lancet. 1962;1:59–63.
22. Jones R, Lovett RW. Orthopedic surgery. New York: Wm Wood & Co.; 1923. p. 549–51.

Chapter 5
Supraclavicular Approach

The supraclavicular approach is the oldest one which attempted to deal with the neurogenic thoracic outlet syndrome, even though removal of a normal first thoracic rib to relieve compression of the brachial plexus was reported earlier by Brickner [1]. The operation begins with a transverse incision made above the clavicle on the affected side. After entering the subcutaneous tissue and dividing the platysma muscle the sternocleidomastoid muscle is then partially divided. Some advocate that the muscle be divided totally in order to expose the posterior space, but others only divide part of the muscle. The posterior space, consisting solely of subcutaneous tissue, is reflected laterally; the external jugular vein does not need to be divided. At the bottom of the space lies the anterior scalene muscle. This is carefully exposed, paying particular attention to protecting the phrenic nerve which runs anterior to the muscle. As the nerve gradually reaches the clavicle it tends to migrate medially towards the mediastinum, thereby separating itself from the muscle. This approach does not allow dissection of the first rib in its entire length. The field does permit the first rib to be visualized in its superior portion anteriorly, but as the dissection is carried out posteriorly it becomes possible to dissect the rib circumferentially. The subclavian vein can now be visualized as it lies exactly in front of the anterior scalene muscle; this vessel must be retracted off the first rib. The course of the vein can be followed towards the mediastinum and then down behind the manubrium of the sternum. Dividing the sternocleidomastoid muscle allows the surgeon to see the junction of the innominate and internal jugular veins, but the portion of innominate vein so exposed which can be isolated is limited.

Since the operation is aimed at relieving arterial and neurogenic compression, the dissection must now be continued posteriorly. The trigone formed by the anterior scalene muscle, the middle scalene muscle, and the superior aspect of the first rib should be clearly identified. After the anterior scalene muscle is divided, the subclavian artery can be seen and retracted superiorly preserving all its branches, particularly the mid cervical branch. The vertebral artery can also be identified originating from the superior aspect of the subclavian. By retracting the subclavian artery superiorly the fibers of the middle scalene muscle can be visualized and divided. Mobilizing the subclavian artery anteriorly, the dissection is continued

J.E. Molina, *New Techniques for Thoracic Outlet Syndromes*,
DOI 10.1007/978-1-4614-5471-7_5, © Springer Science+Business Media New York 2013

posteriorly over the superior aspect of the first rib. All the trunks of the brachial plexus are immediately behind and somewhat superior to the artery. They are now gently retracted in order to expose the remaining rib. Special attention needs to be paid to the long thoracic nerve which crosses over the rib before descending laterally over the rib cage. This must be preserved because it innervates the serratus muscle. The dissection is continued behind the brachial plexus, dividing all the fibers of the middle scalene muscle until the junction of the first rib with the transverse process is reached. By staying close to the periostum of the rib, laceration of the dome of the pleura can be avoided, allowing the entire resection of the first rib and the scalene muscles to be done in an extrapleural manner. At this point, the rib is divided posteriorly at the junction with the transverse process. The rib behind the clavicle is divided at the most anterior point of its exposure. Unfortunately, the most anterior portion of the first rib cannot be removed using this approach unless a subclavicular incision is also made. The supraclavicular approach has been widely used and quite effective in decompressing the brachial plexus and the subclavian artery.

Reference

1. Brickner WM. Brachial plexus pressure by the normal 1st rib. Ann Surg. 1927;85:858–72.

Chapter 6
Transpleural Infraclavicular Approach

This lesser known approach is also used for treatment of the neurogenic-arterial thoracic outlet syndrome. The technique was published by Nelson and Jenson in 1970 [1], and further modified by Murphy et al. in 1980 [2]. The patient must be placed in the lateral decubitus position at 45°. The incision is made in a subclavicular transverse fashion and after separating the fibers of the pectoralis major muscle the first rib is approached. The inferior border of the first rib is then dissected. In order to accomplish visualization and dissection of that rib, the procedure now becomes an intrapleural one (i.e., a limited thoracotomy). The costosternal junction is divided with a rib cutter. Once the anterior end of the first rib is isolated it can be held with a Kocher forceps or a bone holder to facilitate circumferential dissection. By displacement of the rib downward, the anterior scalene muscle is exposed and can be divided at the point of its insertion onto the rib. Further downward displacement of the rib exposes the scalene medius muscle insertion which is also divided. The subclavian vessels are retracted superiorly, while the greater and the lesser curvature of the first rib are now exposed and further dissected until the junction with the transverse process is reached posteriorly. The rib is divided at that level and removed. In the published descriptions of this operation, the posterior end of the rib is best divided using a Sauerbruch rib shear because it is sufficiently narrow to be positioned far posteriorly on the rib very close to its junction with the transverse process.

This approach is essentially a thoracotomy done in the apex of the chest. No further reports concerning it have been published since 1971. It is, however, a feasible operation even though quite cumbersome. One of its disadvantages is obviously that the pleural space is entered, requiring that a chest tube be placed to re-expand the lung and drain any fluid collections postoperatively. Another limitation of this approach is that surgical access to an associated cervical rib or to an abnormal fusion of the first and second rib posteriorly, which occurs occasionally in young people, is inadequate. Additional difficulties of the infraclavicular transpleural approach alone include limitations to perform neurolysis if that becomes necessary and the fact that it is probably not applicable to the treatment of subclavian vein

J.E. Molina, *New Techniques for Thoracic Outlet Syndromes*,
DOI 10.1007/978-1-4614-5471-7_6, © Springer Science+Business Media New York 2013

obstruction because of the lateral decubitous patient position, clearly not as optimal as a supine patient position to address this problem (see treatment of Paget–Schroetter syndrome).

References

1. Nelson RM, Jenson CB. Anterior approach for excision of the first rib surgical technique. Ann Thorac Surg. 1970;9(1):30–5.
2. Murphy TO, Piper CA, Kanar EA, McAlexander RA. Subclavicular approach to first rib resection. Am J Surg. 1980;139:634–6.

Chapter 7
The Paraclavicular Approach to Address Arterial Complications

This technique involves the use of two incisions: one supraclavicular and another infraclavicular. The two-incisions approach above and below the clavicle is successful in exposing the subclavian artery, particularly in patients with a cervical rib in whom the artery has developed a poststenotic aneurysm, and associated thrombosis with peripheral embolism to the arm. To deal with these problems it is necessary to expose the origin of the subclavian artery and to release all the compressing structures of the thoracic outlet by doing a scalenectomy. In addition, exposure of the distal axillary artery is necessary in order to excise the aneurysmal portion of the artery with the thrombus and to implant an interposition graft. In these cases, the addition of a supraclavicular incision is necessary in order to get control of the inflow, at the origin of the subclavian artery. The concurrent occurrence of these problems is relatively rare these days because patients with neurogenic-arterial thoracic outlet syndromes usually seek medical attention before they evolve to this extent. Nevertheless, in our experience we have encountered few such patients, one of whom had a subclavian aneurysm and subsequently developed multiple peripheral emboli to the hand and fingers. That situation required balloon catheter embolectomy of both the brachial and radial arteries which were exposed at the elbow as well as at the wrist level. The patient recovered well without experiencing necrosis of any fingers. The function of the hand recovered completely. In another patient, the aneurysm was removed and replaced with an 8 mm PTFE (Goretex) graft followed by anticoagulation of the patient for 2 months. This patient rethrombosed the graft later but required only subsequent thrombolysis and balloon dilation of the distal anastomosis; the patient recovered and has been asymptomatic for more than 6 years. The importance of obtaining arteriography in cases with abnormal preoperative ultrasounds particularly when a cervical rib is present before undertaking any type of surgery cannot be overemphasized. Fortunately, however most of the time the artery is well preserved and the standard dual approach used by us to remove the 1st rib and the cervical rib solves the entire problem without the need for any direct arterial repair.

J.E. Molina, *New Techniques for Thoracic Outlet Syndromes*,
DOI 10.1007/978-1-4614-5471-7_7,

Chapter 8
The Transaxillary Alone Approach for Removal of the First Rib

For many years, the need to resect the first rib was the only accepted approach to decompressing the thoracic outlet. However, McCleery [1] suggested that scalenectomy alone was sufficient. Accumulated experience proved this to be ineffective reinforcing the need to remove the rib. In 1966 Roos [2] designed the technique now called the transaxillary approach which allows the transection of the anterior as well as the middle scalene muscles and resection of the rib to accomplish a complete decompression of the posterior thoracic outlet, all done through an incision that is not visible from the front or the back. Since that time the operation has been performed frequently by many thoracic surgeons primarily to treat the neurogenic-arterial thoracic outlet syndrome for which this operation was principally designed.

The method requires that at operation the arm of the patient be abducted 90° away from the chest wall [3–5]. An incision is made transversely below the hairline between the posterior border of the pectoralis major muscle and the anterior border of the latissimus dorsi (Fig. 8.1). The incision is carried down through the subcutaneous tissue until the rib cage is reached. From there, the dissection progresses up towards the apex of the chest until the first rib is exposed, and the structures above that level, primarily the subclavian vein, are visualized and retracted to prevent their injury. The incision also exposes the anterior scalene muscle inserting on top of the first rib and exposes part of the medial scalene muscle. Subperiosteal dissection of the first rib is accomplished inferiorly. The anterior scalene muscle is visualized behind the subclavian vein and in front of the subclavian artery. It is easily divided, freeing up the entire area between the two vessels. Retracting the neurovascular bundle gently, division of the first rib is carried out anteriorly and ideally, as far posterior as the junction between the first rib and the vertebral transverse process. At that level the rib is divided and removed from the field. Herein lies a major problem with this approach.

The entire operation is done through the incision described; unfortunately it offers a very limited space not only to maneuver and separate the structures but also to position the rib cutter instruments properly. They are quite bulky, and difficult to utilize in this area. Although large series have been reported [5–9] with satisfactory results, these limitations have contributed to a significant number of complications leading to

J.E. Molina, *New Techniques for Thoracic Outlet Syndromes*,
DOI 10.1007/978-1-4614-5471-7_8, © Springer Science+Business Media New York 2013

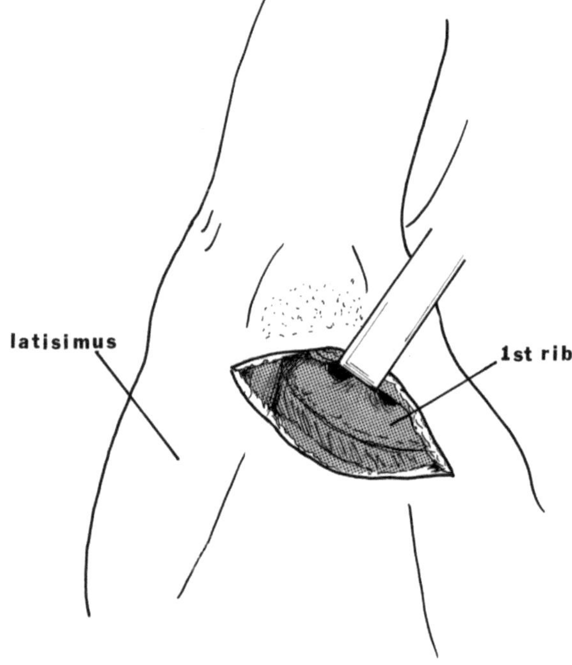

Fig. 8.1 Through the axillary incision the rib cage is reached. The adipose tissue is retracted superiorly and the first rib is exposed first by palpation and then by dissection lifting the subclavian vein away from the superior surface of the first rib

neurogenic damage, vascular injuries, and bleeding. All of these have been reported by several authors including Dale [10], Mellière [11], and Horowitz [12]. Theoretically the rib is ideally divided flush with its sternal insertion. Even though the operation is supposed to remove the entire rib, however, this objective is rarely achieved, particularly in muscular individuals in which retraction of the pectoralis major muscle anteriorly is necessary to reach the point of insertion of the rib into the sternum. Consequently, the surgeon often divides the first rib at some distance from this point [13–16] leaving a residual stump anteriorly. This is often true at the posterior stump as well, because it is impossible, occasionally, to reach all the way back to the junction between the rib and the transverse process (Fig. 8.2). If the patient does not suffer concomitant venous obstruction, leaving an anterior stump of the first rib probably does not matter as long as the posterior half of the rib is removed. Another disadvantage exists. During the operation the arm must be held in 90° of abduction, and this poses a mechanical physical problem. Initially an assistant was suggested to hold the arm upwards [2, 3, 17] while the surgeon conducted the operation, giving no opportunity to the surgical assistant to see what was being done during the hour or more needed to accomplish the entire operation. The assistant invariably gets tired while holding the arm in the needed position, particularly in large individuals or obese people, making the whole procedure very cumbersome and disjointed. In order to overcome these limitations several mechanical solutions have been implemented designed to replace the assistant entirely with a more reliable and steady exposure while preserving the possibilities of elevating or lowering the arm as needed. In our institution, we recommend exclusively the dual approach described further ahead.

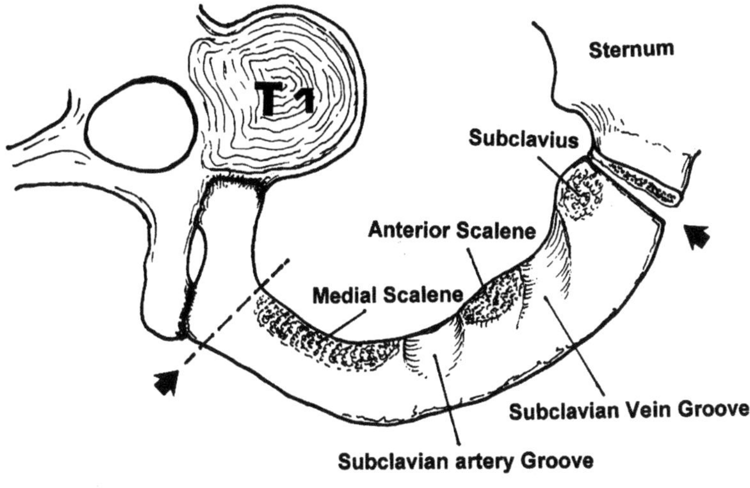

Fig. 8.2 Superior view of the first rib showing (*arrows*) the level at which the first rib should be divided for removal in cases with neurogenic thoracic outlet syndrome. Sites of muscle insertions are depicted

That includes a transaxillary stage and for which we utilize a mechanical device [18], which attaches to the table and allows for elevation of the arm at 90° by using a crank provided with this device (Fig. 8.3). However, we use this device only as part of our dual approach technique described in the dual approach section.

Complications Doing the Transaxillary Approach

As noted, there have been many reports over the past 25 years detailing problems and complications using the transaxillary approach to first rib resection. These include vascular injuries; neurologic injuries to the trunks of the brachial plexus, hemothorax, pneumothorax, and areas of anesthesia; or numbness of indeterminate nature along the chest wall or the inner aspect of the arm postoperatively. Dale [10] surveyed 259 thoracic surgeons who regularly perform this operation. He found 102 cases of paralysis, 2 of them permanent, and 171 of them partial, and vascular injuries to the subclavian artery requiring emergent vascular procedures to repair and to control bleeding and hematomas in the area. In addition Mellière [11] reported on the experience of 66 surgeons familiar with the operation who noted lacerations of the subclavian artery requiring reoperation often involving a formal thoracotomy to repair the vessel. These included four cases of complete transection of the artery doing the removal of the rib which necessitated implant of a vascular graft, as well as injuries to the internal mammary artery and, in four cases, damage to the subclavian vein, the repair of which was always described as extremely difficult. They also described brachial plexus injuries including

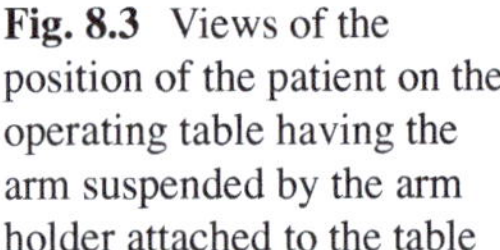

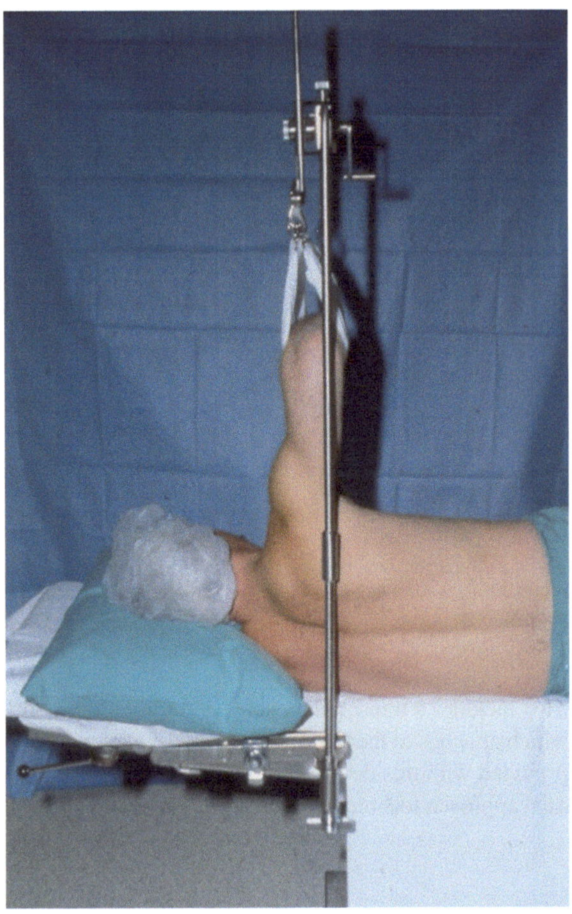

Fig. 8.3 Views of the position of the patient on the operating table having the arm suspended by the arm holder attached to the table

complete division of the nerves caused by the bone-cutting instrument resulting in two cases of permanent paralysis of the arm, and nine cases of scapula alata, the "winged scapula," four of which were permanent. They observed five cases of phrenic nerve paralysis and other miscellaneous injuries including paralysis of the deltoid muscle and cases of Horner syndrome, and also a few cases of lymphatic vessel injuries with formation of lymphoceles and occasionally chylothorax. Horowitz [12] also reported multiple brachial plexus injuries with causalgia using this approach.

As explained above, several reasons exist which can cause these injuries. First the area of exposure needed to visualize these structures from the subaxillary incision all the way up to the level of the first rib is very limited. Damage to the surrounding structures can also occur when the bone-cutting instrument is introduced. These instruments are large, bulky, and do not allow for clear visualization of the instrument tips, so that they can easily catch soft tissue structures like the vein, the artery, or the nerves. The Roos Rib cutter in particular is so large that it sometimes is impossible to position it properly particularly in small individuals.

Other instruments like the Giertz-Stille are somewhat narrower and easier to control particularly but too short in a deep small area. Other injuries occur while using sharp instruments, mostly scissors. Less serious complications like the occurrence of pneumothorax can be totally avoided following the proper steps as explained under the dual approach. The simple maneuver of stripping the periosteum off of the inferior surface of the first rib first, creating an extrapleural space, prevents pneumothorax when the anterior scalene muscle is divided.

Other limitations of this approach include, as already noted, the inability to reach the most posterior end of the rib before dividing it, thus leaving a stump. This results in recurrence of the symptoms weeks or months later, often requiring reoperation. It is my belief that the transaxillary approach alone is frequently not sufficient to obtain a complete release of the compression to the brachial plexus or the artery. Therefore as explained previously a dual approach is always used by us to attain excellent exposure and prevent complications. It has additional advantages.

Urschel has addressed the problem of recurrent symptoms following transaxillary resection of the first rib. [13, 14] When these patients need to be reoperated he has used what is called the posterior approach. As described by Clagett [19] and others [4, 6, 20] this involves a very formidable operation necessitating division of several muscles of the back. We believe that all of these inconveniences can be overcome by using the dual approach.

It has been suggested that the long-term results of an operation aimed to relieve the compression of the brachial plexus must be evaluated at the minimum time of 18 months [21]. Some of the patients, following this operation, feel immediate relief and change in their symptoms. However it takes several weeks for the edema to disappear and for them to feel the benefits of the decompression. Because most of the failures or recurrences occur within 12 months [21] it is critical to maintain communication with patients for at least a year, particularly if the operation performed utilized only the transaxillary incision. This is so, because the chances for symptomatic recurrence are greater if the rib has not been completely removed, thereby leaving a stump posteriorly with part of the middle scalene muscles intact. Treatment of recurrent symptoms is described later.

References

1. McCleery RS, Kersterson JE, Kirtley JA, Love RB. Subclavius and anterior scalene muscle compression as a cause of intermittent obstruction of the subclavian vein. Ann Surg. 1951;133:588–602.
2. Roos DB. Transaxillary approach for first rib resection to relieve thoracic outlet syndrome. Ann Surg. 1966;163:354–8.
3. Valentine RJ, Wind CG. Anatomic exposures in vascular surgery. Philadelphia: Lippincott Williams & Wilkins; 2003.
4. Urschel Jr HC, Cooper JD. Atlas of thoracic surgery. New York: Churchill Livingston; 1995.
5. Urschel Jr HC, Patel AN. Chapter 123. Thoracic outlet syndromes. In: Sugarbaker DJ, editor. Adult chest surgery. New York: McGraw Hill; 2009. p. 1024–33.

6. Mackinnon S, Patterson GA, Urschel Jr. HC. Ch 52: Thoracic outlet syndromes. In: F. Griffith Pearson, editor. Thoracic surgery. 2nd ed. New York: Churchill Livingston; 2002. p. 1393–415.
7. Urschel Jr HC, Razzuk MA. Chapter 18: Thoracic outlet syndrome. In: Sabiston DC, Spencer F, editors. Surgery of the chest. 5th ed. Philadelphia: Saunders; 1990. p. 536–53.
8. Sander RJ, Pearse WH. The treatment of thoracic outlet syndrome: a comparison of different operations. J Vasc Surg. 1989;10:626–34.
9. Urschel Jr HC, Razzuk MA. Neurovascular compression in the thoracic outlet: changing management over 50 years. Ann Surg. 1998;228:609–17.
10. Dale A. Thoracic outlet compression syndrome. Critique in 1982. Arch Surg. 1982;117: 1437–46.
11. Mellière D, Becquemin J-P, Etienne G, Le Cheviller B. Severe injuries resulting from operations for thoracic outlet syndrome: can they be avoided? J Cardiovasc Surg. 1991;32: 599–603.
12. Horowitz SH. Brachial plexus injuries with causalgia resulting from transaxillary rib resection. Arch Surg. 1985;120:1189–91.
13. Urschel Jr HC, Razzuk MA. The failed operation for thoracic outlet syndrome: the difficulty of diagnosis and management. Ann Thorac Surg. 1986;42:523–8.
14. Urschel Jr HC, Razzuk MA, Albers JE, Wood RE, Paulson DL. Reoperations for recurrent thoracic outlet syndrome. Ann Thorac Surg. 1976;21:19–25.
15. Cheng SWK, Stoney RJ. Supraclavicular reoperation for neurogenic thoracic outlet syndrome. J Vasc Surg. 1994;19:565–72.
16. Sanders RJ, Haug CE, Pearce WH. Recurrent thoracic outlet syndrome. J Vasc Surg. 1990; 12:390–400.
17. Wood VE, Twito R, Verska JM. Thoracic outlet syndrome. The results of first rib resection in 100 patients. Orthop Clin North Am. 1988;19:131–46.
18. Molina JE. Combined posterior and transaxillary approach for neurogenic thoracic outlet syndrome. J Am Coll Surg. 1998;187:39–45.
19. Clagett OT. Research and prosearch. Presidential Address. J Thorac Cardiovasc Surg. 1962;44:153–66.
20. Ferguson TB, Burford TH, Roper CL. Neurovascular compression at the superior thoracic aperture. Surgical management. Ann Surg. 1968;167:573–9.
21. Altobelli GG, Kudo T, Haas BT, Chandra FA, Moy JL, Ahn SS. Thoracic outlet syndrome: pattern of clinical success after operative decompression. J Vasc Surg. 2005;42:122–8.

Chapter 9
The Posterior Approach

In 1962 the posterior approach to the removal of the first rib was proposed by Clagett [1] which he believed gave better access to its posterior end. It is a formidable operation based on thoracoplasty incisions with which the surgeons of the day were very familiar because of its use to treat pulmonary tuberculosis. The operation involved removal of the ribs in order to create a soft tissue collapse over the upper lobe of the lung to promote healing of the tuberculous process. That operation involves a long vertical posterior incision that divides the trapezius, the serratus, and the rhomboid muscles with retraction of the scapula laterally in order to expose the rib cage. Leffert [2] points out that, with respect to the thoracic outlet syndrome, this approach is very bloody and cuts through precisely those muscles one is trying to rehabilitate. Urschel [3] recommended it be used only when an inadequately resected portion of the first rib remains after previous attempt to relieve recurrent symptoms.

Occasionally the operation is done in very obese patients because in the judgment of the surgeon, it might be safer to approach the problem from the back rather than through the transaxillary or the supraclavicular route. An additional risk of dividing all the muscles of the back is the possibility of causing injury to the elevator of the scapula, leaving the patient with an additional disability postoperatively. In general, therefore, the posterior approach is not used routinely for removal of the first rib to decompress the brachial plexus or the subclavian artery. Ferguson [4] made the observation that, even though carrying the incision around the tip of the scapula allows this shoulder girdle to be displaced anteriorly, resection of the first rib alone is still difficult. Therefore, he felt that initially a segment of the second rib should also be removed subperiostically in order to reach the first rib. He reported good results in 12 patients with a follow-up of up to 56 months. The general objection to this technique is nevertheless the same: the extensive operation of obligatory transaction of so many muscles in the back. Much of this can be avoided by using other techniques like the combined approach of a transaxillary and a transverse limited posterior incision over the trapezius, as described by us in 1998 [5] without sacrificing any muscles.

J.E. Molina, *New Techniques for Thoracic Outlet Syndromes*,
DOI 10.1007/978-1-4614-5471-7_9,

References

1. Clagett OT. Research and prosearch. Presidential address. J Thorac Cardiovasc Surg. 1962;44:153–66.
2. Leffert RD. Thoracic outlet syndromes. Hand Clin. 1992;8:285–97.
3. Mackinnon S, Patterson GA, Urschel Jr. HC. Thoracic outlet syndromes Ch 52. In: Thoracic surgery. 2nd ed. Ch 52. Churchill Livingston Publishers New York, Edingburgh, London, Philadelphia; 2002. p. 1393–1415.
4. Ferguson TB, Burford TH, Roper CL. Neurovascular compression at the superior thoracic aperture. Surgical management. Ann Surg. 1968;167:573–9.
5. Molina JE. Combined posterior and transaxillary approach for neurogenic thoracic outlet syndrome. J Am Coll Surg. 1998;187:39–45.

Chapter 10
The New Dual Approach

The Dual Approach for resection of the first rib was created because of the necessity to take advantage of the transaxillary route to reach the anterior portion of the rib while at the same time avoiding the multiple complications that can occur when trying to use that approach alone to reach the posterior end of the rib. It is, therefore, a combination of a transaxillary and a new posterior incision very different from the vertical incision proposed by Clagett and used by Urschel, and others. This new technique was first published in 1998 [1] and has been used for more than 25 years at the University of Minnesota for specific elective treatment of the neurogenic thoracic outlet syndrome when no vascular repair needs to be undertaken in the subclavian artery. It is our standard operation for the uncomplicated neurogenic-arterial thoracic outlet syndrome.

The operation consists of making an incision in the subaxillary area between the anterior border of the latissimus dorsi and lateral border of the pectoralis major muscle (Fig. 8.1). In order to avoid the difficulties inherent in having an assistant hold the arm at 90° abduction from the chest wall throughout the entire case, a new device was also developed in order to have the arm automatically held in this position. This new device has the added capability of using a crank system to increase or decrease the amount of traction applied (Figs. 8.3 and 10.1) we think this device is more practical than the pulley system devised by Urschel [2]. In addition to the arm holder, an "omnitrack" system is attached to the table on the opposite side in the front of the patient with a single-angled rod to which a retractor blade can be attached. This retracts the pectoralis major muscle anteriorly allowing the surgeon to reach as much as possible the anterior end of the rib attached to the sternum. This device and the Omnitrack system are used only for implementation of the transaxillary stage of the dual approach. The dissection accomplished using this system enables dissection of the first rib from the front to the level where the subclavian artery crosses the rib laterally. This is not a totally adequate incision to remove the subclavius tendon, which is far anterior. At best this tendon can be divided in part but not resected. The anterior scalene muscle can occasionally be plainly visualized before the rib is divided; more often, especially in muscular individuals, the rib needs to be divided anteriorly first in order to expose the entire anterior scalene muscle. This can then be divided and dissection continued laterally to divide at least half of the fibers of the medial scalene muscle without exert-

J.E. Molina, *New Techniques for Thoracic Outlet Syndromes*,
DOI 10.1007/978-1-4614-5471-7_10,

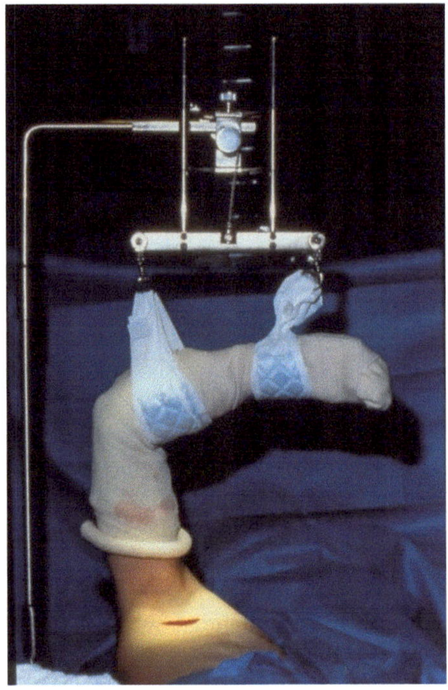

Fig. 10.1 Operative photograph of the arm holder in operation exposing the axillary area where the transverse incision is made to approach the first rib

ing unusual traction on the neurovascular bundle containing the brachial plexus and the subclavian artery. This is accomplished using the omnitrack blade. After completing the transaxillary stage, the second approach of the dual technique is then undertaken. The arm is taken down from the arm holder and positioned along the patient's body. Attention is now directed to the back of the neck and shoulder.

The posterior incision is made parallel to the trapezius ridge about 2 cm behind this border running from the midline of the spine towards the shoulder (Fig. 10.2). The trapezius muscle fibers are not transected, but only separated or split in their direction and the rest of the exposure is achieved by retracting the elevator of the scapular muscle laterally.

Operative Technique Details

The patient is positioned in the lateral decubitus over a bean bag which is activated by applying continuous suction until it becomes hard and immobilizes the patient in this position. The patient's arm is prepped in the operative field held by an IV pole with a Velcro padded bracelet that allows the arm to be suspended for the prep solution. The antiseptic scrub and paint are applied to the chest to be operated and to the arm up to the middle of the forearm. A split drape is placed covering the lower body, except for the arm. At that point the arm is taken down from the IV pole holding strap, wrapped with a sterile impervious sleeve secured with an ace bandage and brought down to lie

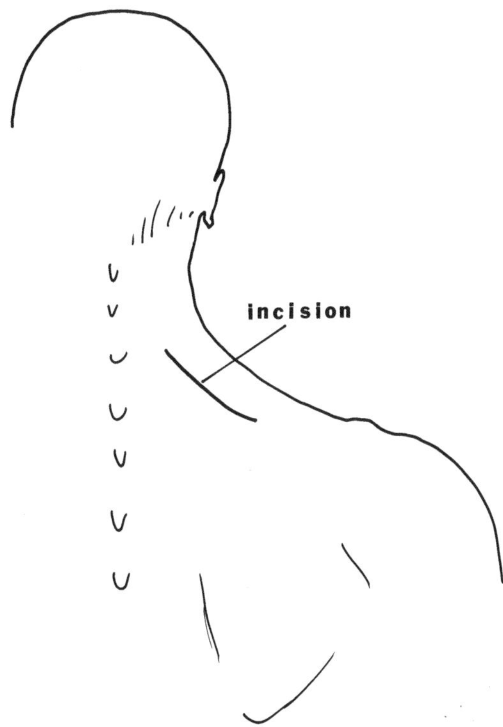

Fig. 10.2 Site of the posterior incision made behind the trapezius ridge to approach the posterior end of the first rib as well as the cervical rib insertion on the spine

along the patient's body while a second split drape is placed covering the head in a reverse fashion to meet the other split drape which has been placed from the lower part of the body. In this way, the arm is completely sterile in the operative field.

At this point the arm holder is attached to the table as shown in Figs. 8.3 and 10.1. Using sterile slings the forearm of the patient is placed on the horizontal lifting section of the arm holder, which will keep the arm steady at 90° in abduction while retaining the ability to raise it as needed.

As in the transaxillary technique, the usual incision is made below the hairline of the axilla transversally between the pectoralis major muscle and the latissimus dorsi (Fig. 8.1). The dissection continues through the subcutaneous tissue to reach the rib cage. From here the dissection is carried up using the cautery towards the apex of the chest. As we reach the first rib and the subclavian vein is visualized, the Omnitrack automatic retractor is installed onto the table in front. It is fitted with a single-angled bar where a blade is attached to it to retract the pectoralis major muscle anteriorly. Once satisfactory exposure is obtained in this manner, the surgeon proceeds to detach the subclavian vein from the top of the first rib. The area contains only loose connective tissue that can be handled easily using the cautery. In the majority of cases once the vein is identified going into the mediastinum the anterior scalene muscle tendon can be visualized behind it. At this point it is not advisable to try to divide the anterior scalene muscle, because frequently the dome of the pleura abuts this structure, and dissection done behind the

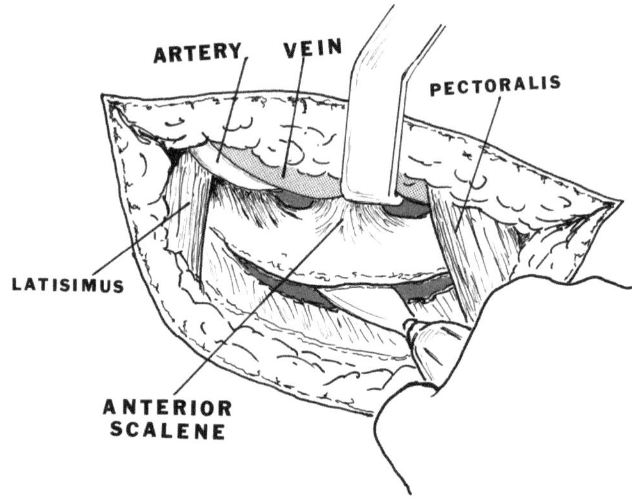

Fig. 10.3 This shows the second step using the transaxillary approach to remove the first rib. Subperiosteal dissection is carried out of the inferior surface of the first rib. Division of the anterior scalene muscle is postponed after an extrapleural space is created

muscle tendon may create a tear in the pleura, collapse of the lung, and the need to place a chest tube. Therefore, at this point the proper second step is to make an incision along the inferior border of the first rib using the cautery followed by utilizing the periosteal elevator to detach the periosteum from the inferior surface of the rib from the front to as far back as the instrument can reach (Fig. 10.3). The maneuver creates an extrapleural space into which a finger can be easily inserted to detach the pleura bluntly from the rib (Fig. 10.4). The tendon of the anterior scalene muscle can now be safely hooked with the right-angle clamp, and divided (Fig. 10.5). All fibers should be divided from the front to the back, and using digital manipulation the surgeon can verify that the entire rib is free of any further attachments. There is no danger of injuring the phrenic nerve because at that level the nerve has already migrated separating its course from the scalene muscle more medial towards the mediastinum.

In some cases, when the chest configuration is more cylindrical than conical, the first rib is also difficult to visualize because of the protrusion of the second rib. This may make safe division of the anterior scalene muscle impossible even after creating the extra pleural space described above. Manual pressure must be applied to the second rib by the surgeon to reach the inferior edge of the first rib. This problem is sometimes predictable by observing the lateral outline silhouette of the rib cage on plain X-rays. The patients who have a more cylindrical type of chest up to the second rib have at that point a sudden or sharp angulation towards the first rib, instead of the more usual conical or pyramidal shape of the entire rib cage (Fig. 10.6).

In this instance, division of the rib anteriorly greatly facilitates the exposure of the tendon of the anterior scalene muscle because once the rib is freed anteriorly, exerting manual downward pressure on the free end of the rib exposes the area of

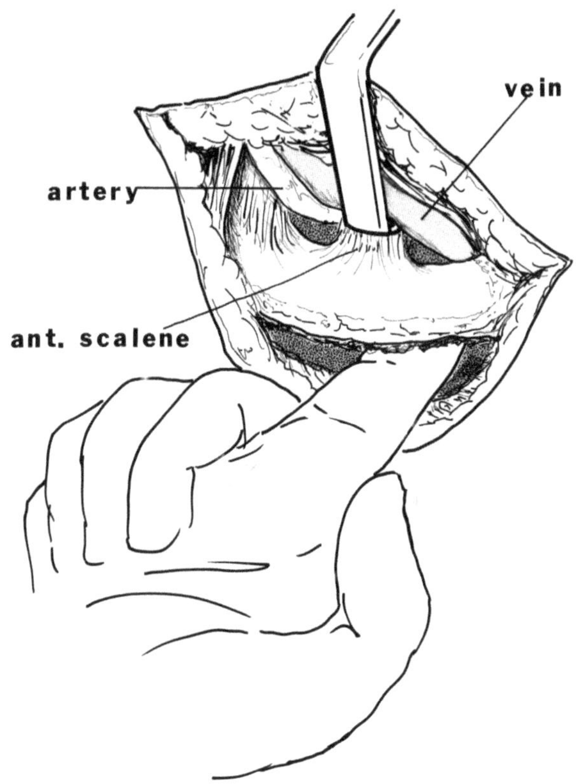

Fig. 10.4 Following creation of the extrapleural space then with a digital maneuver the remaining of the pleura is detached from the inferior surface of the first rib. The vessels are retracted superiorly in order to expose the anterior scalene muscle tendon

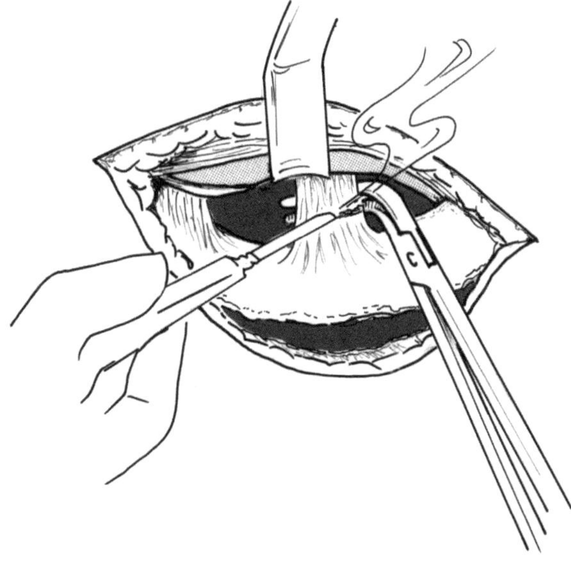

Fig. 10.5 After creating the extrapleural space to prevent pneumothorax a right-angle forceps is passed around the base of the anterior scalene muscle tendon and divided with the cautery close to its insertion on the rib

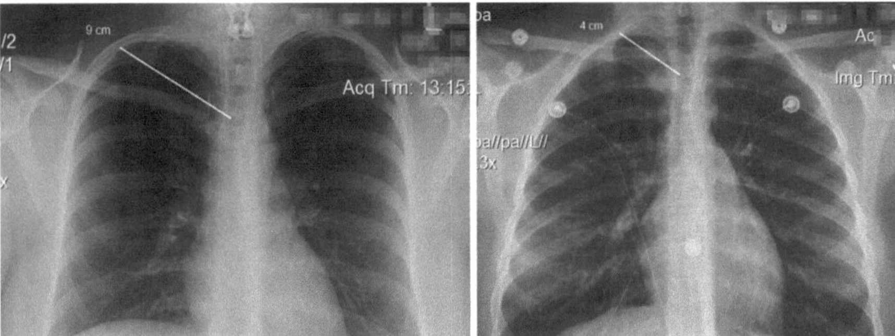

Fig. 10.6 Chest X-rays of two patients showing different upper ribs anatomic configuration. (**a**) TOS patient. Cylindrical type of chest showing prominent arch of the second rib. This setting obstructs the view of the first rib when a transaxillary route is used. Notice the distance from the sternal notch to the arch of the second rib of 9 cm. (**b**) Normal asymptomatic patient. A conical smooth configuration between the second and first rib. Distance from the arch of the second rib to the sternal notch is only 4 cm

the anterior scalene muscle, which at this moment can be divided. The dissection is now carried back towards the middle scalene muscle, which can be exposed by retracting superiorly the neurovascular bundle containing the subclavian artery and the brachial plexus (Fig. 10.7). The fibers of the middle scalene muscle inserting on the top of the rib can be divided using the cautery as far back as feasible, but it is better to try to divide as much as possible to facilitate the second stage of the operation. No attempt is made to reach the posterior end of the rib at this point to prevent any possible injury to the neurovascular bundle. With the above maneuver, the first stage of the operation is complete. The entire area is then irrigated with antibiotic solution and the arm is taken down from the arm holder and laid along the patient's body. All the retractors attached to the table are removed.

The posterior second stage of the operation of this dual approach is now undertaken. The patient is placed into reverse Trendelenburg to facilitate exposure of the region. The posterior incision is made from the midline parallel to the trapezius ridge towards the shoulder (Fig. 10.2). After entering the subcutaneous tissue, the trapezius muscle fibers are encountered and are split in their direction until the retromuscular space is reached. Here the only muscle present that needs to be retracted is the elevator of the scapula. Retracting it is a very important maneuver because the long thoracic nerve runs along its lateral border. To protect it dissection is directed along the medial border of this muscle close to the spine. Using a retractor, the muscle is separated laterally and the first rib, which lays superiorly, is clearly seen as well as the fibers of the medial scalene muscle inserting on top of it (Fig. 10.8). These as well as the intercostal muscles going to the second rib inferiorly are all divided using the cautery. Occasionally fibers of the posterior scalene muscle that normally insert on the top of the second rib interfere with the exposure and some of them may be divided. Most of the time however the posterior scalene muscle is left intact. Once the superior and inferior borders of the first rib are isolated, the dissection is

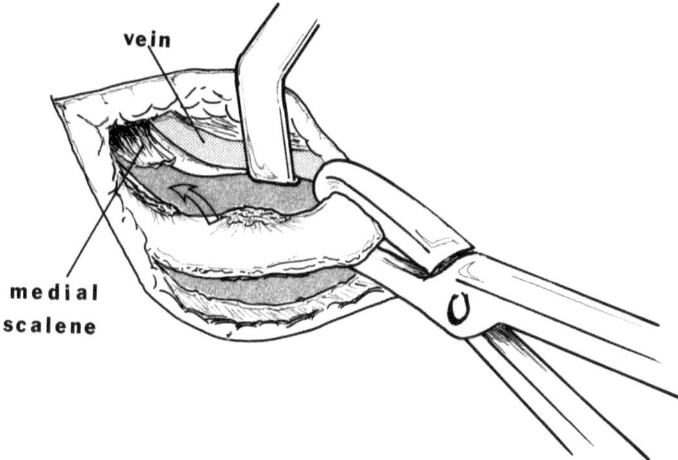

Fig. 10.7 After the anterior scalene muscle is divided the fibers of the medial scalene muscle are also divided detaching it from the superior aspect of the first rib as far back as feasible. The vessels are retracted superiorly and the pleura remains intact. The rib is divided anteriorly

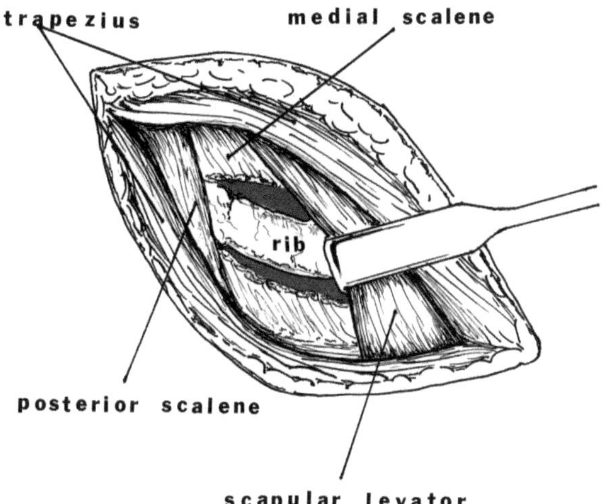

Fig. 10.8 The trapezius muscle has been spread. The scapular elevator muscle has been retracted laterally and the fibers of the medial scalene muscle are incised from the top of the first rib. The intercostal muscle at the inferior border of the first rib is also divided and the extrapleural space is created prior to division of the first rib

continued towards the spine until we reach the joint between the first rib and the transverse process of the vertebral body. A groove can always be palpated at that junction and this is entered also, using the cautery. This marks the level at which the rib will be divided. With blunt digital dissection, the space created above and below the first rib is continued anteriorly to join the extrapleural space already created from the transaxillary dissection. This is easily done and a few remaining fibers attaching

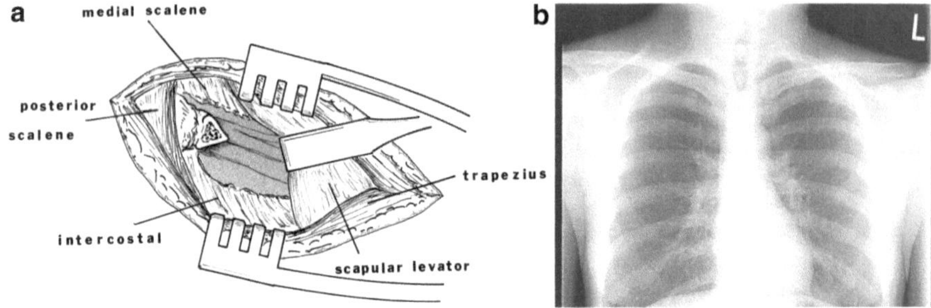

Fig. 10.9 (**a**) Posteriorly the first rib is divided at the junction with the transverse process of the spine and removed from the field. The brachial plexus trunks lay in the extrapleural space over the intact pleura. (**b**) Typical correct resection of the first rib with no residual stump on the right side

to the top of the first rib can also be divided using the cautery while the trapezius and the elevator of the scapular muscle are being retracted. It is important to make sure that no soft tissue remains attached to the bone and to verify that a sufficient extrapleural space has been created along the inner curvature of the rib. This prevents any possible damage to the brachial plexus that must remain in continuity with the pleura away from the rib. Once this is accomplished the rib is divided using the rib cutter at the joint between the rib and the transverse process (Fig. 10.9). The rib is removed from the field, and the area is irrigated with antibiotic solution. Any bleeding is controlled with the use of the cautery. The incision is now closed. The fibers of the trapezius muscle are reapproximated with nonabsorbable material, the subcutaneous tissue is closed with absorbable suture in a running fashion, and the skin is sealed off with Dermabond. We now direct attention back to the subaxillary incision. A Jackson-Pratt drain, or a Blake drain size 19 is laid in the extrapleura space and brought out through a separate incision in the lower part of the chest. The drain is secured to the skin with a stick tie ligature, and connected to a bulb suction system. The subaxillary incision is now closed, the subcutaneous fascia with a running absorbable material followed by either a subdermic or a subcuticular suture, and the skin is sealed off with Dermabond. The estimated total blood loss for the procedure is usually 20 cc or less.

Our dual approach operation offers the following advantages: (a) Avoids neurologic complications; (b) prevents vascular injuries; (c) eliminates the difficulty of reaching the posterior end of the rib; (d) accomplishes complete removal of the rib, therefore preventing reoperation; and finally (e) is cosmetically acceptable.

References

1. Molina JE. Combined posterior and transaxillary approach for neurogenic thoracic outlet syndrome. J Am Coll Surg. 1998;187:39–45.
2. Urschel Jr HC, Razzuk MA. Ch 18. Thoracic outlet syndrome. In: Sabiston DC, Spencer F, editors. Surgery of the chest. 5th ed. Philadelphia: Saunders; 1990. p. 536–53.

Chapter 11
Reoperations for Recurrence of Neurogenic Symptoms

Urschel [1, 2] and collaborators have emphasized the difficulties inherent in treating patients with recurrent symptoms after an initial operation for neurogenic thoracic outlet syndrome. Usually, recurrence is the result of incomplete removal of the first rib during the first operation, a common finding seen on plain X-ray studies. Occasionally it is just a short stump; other times it is a longer segment in which the periosteum of the excised rib has regenerated causing the problem. Incomplete removal of the first rib is a common occurrence in cases operated using the transaxillary approach because of the difficulties encountered in exposing the posterior distal end of the rib. This in turn leads the surgeon to divide the rib at some distance from its origin with the transverse process, resulting in recurrent symptoms. Conversely, if the rib is completely excised during the first operation, recurrent symptoms are unlikely. Accordingly, it is very important during the first operation to achieve complete removal of the rib. The two approaches that have shown to be most effective in this regard are the supraclavicular approach [3, 4] and the combined approach as described by us [5] (i.e., using the transaxillary approach for the anterior portion of the rib and then a limited posterior incision along the trapezius ridge to reach the posterior end of the rib). Removal of residual posterior end of the rib has been also approached using what is called the posterior route, as introduced by Clagget [6] and used by others [1]. As previously noted, this is a very formidable operation requiring division of several muscles. It may also still pose difficulties of visualizing the rib for which Ferguson [7] proposed removal also of the second rib in order to reach the first adequately. This is very tedious and difficult because of the fibrosis that invariably encases the nerve trunks and the subclavian artery. For these reasons, my personal recommendation for removal of the posterior residual stump of the first rib is to use a limited incision parallel to the trapezius ridge which allows the surgeon to approach the top of the residual rib and remove it without risk of injuries to either artery or brachial plexus.

The more difficult problem to solve is what to do if the patient returns again with recurrent symptoms, and there is no residual stump remaining. Attempts of an

J.E. Molina, *New Techniques for Thoracic Outlet Syndromes*,
DOI 10.1007/978-1-4614-5471-7_11, © Springer Science+Business Media New York 2013

operative correction are rarely indicated or successful. The only procedure to be attempted is to remove scar tissue or accomplish a neurolysis [2, 8]. Discomfort may be helped by physical therapy or by a pain clinic management, but none of the methods are totally effective, so some of these unfortunate patients remain symptomatic permanently.

References

1. Urschel Jr HC, Razzuk MA. The failed operation for thoracic outlet syndrome: the difficulty of diagnosis and management. Ann Thorac Surg. 1986;42:523–8.
2. Urschel Jr HC, Razzuk MA, Albers JE, Wood RE, Paulson DL. Reoperations for recurrent thoracic outlet syndrome. Ann Thorac Surg. 1976;21:19–25.
3. Molina JE. Combined Posterior and transaxillary approach for neurogenic thoracic outlet syndrome. J Am Coll Surg. 1998;187:39–45.
4. Altobelli GG, Kudo T, Haas BT, Chandra FA, Moy JL, Ahn SS. Thoracic outlet syndrome: pattern of clinical success after operative decompression. J Vasc Surg. 2005;42:122–8.
5. Quarfordt PG, Ehrenfeld WK, Stoney RJ. Supraclavicular radical scalenectomy and transaxillary first rib resection for thoracic outlet syndrome. A combined approach. Am J Surg. 1984;148:111–6.
6. Clagett OT. Research and prosearch. Presidential Address. J Thorac Cardiovasc Surg. 1962;44:153–66.
7. Ferguson TB, Burford TH, Roper CL. Neurovascular compression at the superior thoracic aperture. Surgical management. Ann Surg. 1968;167:573–9.
8. Cheng SWK, Stoney RJ. Supraclavicular reoperation for neurogenic thoracic outlet syndrome. J Vasc Surg. 1994;19:565–72.

Part II
Venous Thoracic Outlet Syndrome (Paget-Schroetter)

Chapter 12
Symptoms and Physical Findings

The Paget–Schroetter syndrome refers to a sudden thrombosis of the subclavian vein, which is usually associated with physical exertion of the arm due to the patient's occupation or sport activities (Fig. 12.1). The name of the syndrome was given by the physicians who described this syndrome, namely, Paget in England and Von Schroetter in Austria [1–3]. Hughes must be credited with bringing this entity to the clinical knowledge and to label it most properly as we know it today [4, 5]. Typically the patient affected with acute thrombosis of the subclavian vein presents her/himself to the emergency room or to the physician's office complaining of sudden pain in the affected arm as well as swelling and some bluish discoloration of the entire arm. Most often this episode is associated following a sudden effort with the arm. Occasionally the patient has had several episodes in the past that have resolved spontaneously with rest, until finally a very acute severe event takes place that prompts the patient to seek medical attention. The syndrome usually affects young people leading active and productive lives. The occurrence of thrombosis of the vein is often directly related to their occupation or sports activity. Among the sports leading to cause this syndrome are swimming, climbing, weight lifting, tennis playing, and others. Occupations that may lead to the occurrence of this syndrome vary, but usually affects laborers involved in strenuous physical activity with their arms with repetitive movements particularly over the head maneuvers. The physical findings at the time of the examination show usually severe edema of the arm particularly between the elbow and the shoulder, but it may also involve the forearm and the hand and fingers (Fig. 12.2a, b). The entire upper extremity may have bluish discoloration along with this edema. The radial pulse usually is always present and there are no signs of ischemia.

J.E. Molina, *New Techniques for Thoracic Outlet Syndromes*,
DOI 10.1007/978-1-4614-5471-7_12,

DIE

ANGEBORENEN HERZKRANKHEITEN.

VON

PROF. DR. HERMANN VIERORDT

IN TÜBINGEN.

ERKRANKUNGEN DES HERZBEUTELS.

VON

PROF. L. v. SCHRÖTTER

IN WIEN.

ERKRANKUNGEN DER GEFÄSSE.

VON

PROF. L. v. SCHRÖTTER

IN WIEN.

Fig. 12.1 Original report by Schroetter in 1884

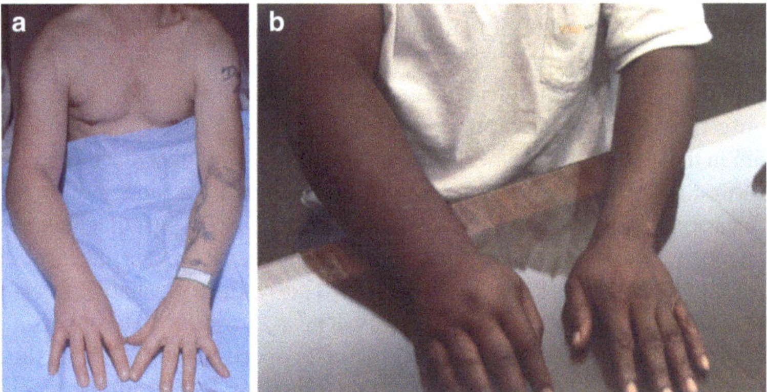

Fig. 12.2 (**a**) Typical aspect of the acute event of subclavian vein effort thrombosis in the right arm. The patient was seen within 5 days of the occurrence. Significant edema can be appreciated in comparison with the left arm which is normal. (**b**) Another patient after 2 years of chronic obstruction

References

1. Paget J. Clinical Lectures and Essays. London 1875. Longmans Green & Co. Huges ESR Venous Obstruction in the upper extremity. Brit J Surg 1948;36:155–163.
2. Schroetter VL. Erkranlungen der Gefasse. Northnagel Handbuch der Pathologie und Therapie. Wien: Alfred Holder edit; 1884.
3. Schrötter L. Erkrankungen der Gefässe: in Spezielle Pathologie und Therapie. Wien: Alfred Hölder; 1901. p. 491–534.
4. Hughes ESR. Venous obstruction in the upper extremity (Paget-Schroetter's syndrome). Int Abstracts of Surg 1949;88:89–127.
5. Hughes ESR. Venous obstruction in the upper extremity. Brit J Surg. 1948;36(142):155–63.

Chapter 13
Etiology

Obstruction of the Subclavian Vein at the thoracic inlet is caused by compression in a vise mechanism between the tendons of the subclavius muscle and the costal clavicular ligament superiorly, the anterior scalene muscle posteriorly, and the first rib inferiorly (Fig. 13.1a, b). Thrombosis of the vein at that level is generally classified as either acute or chronic. The latter is a consequence of repeated pinching of the vein causing gradual fibrosis of its walls and, ultimately, progressive stenosis. When the process gets to a critical point, the vein finally obstructs causing an acute thrombosis at that level (Fig. 13.2a, b). This may rapidly propagate distally into the axillary vein or even down into the arms. Acute thrombosis on the other hand is due to a sudden unusual effort involving arms which damages the intima of the subclavian vein and precipitates acute thrombosis. The vein usually retains its normal caliber once the clot is removed and the compression mechanism around the vessel is relieved. In the case of recurrent chronic pinching of the vein causing gradual stenosis and fibrosis, the patient develops collateral circulation. Initially this may not be noticeable until total occlusion occurs and the collateral veins around the shoulder and the axillary vein become very prominent very rapidly (Fig. 13.3a, b). The arm may become significantly edematous, and frequently develops a blue hue (Fig. 12.1a, b). The illustration that Von Schroetter displayed in his original contribution [1] shows obvious advanced collateralization, which suggests that the obstruction has been present for a considerable period of time. In our own series of over 200 cases treated, only about 3% were seen during the acute event in a perfectly normal individual with no previous episodes of compression of the vein; the rest presented in the chronic stage of the obstruction. We call the thrombosis acute if this condition is diagnosed within the first 2 weeks of the original occurrence; beyond 2 weeks we consider the thrombosis chronic because we have seen some patients even within that period of time who presented with total fibrotic obliteration of the vein extending distally into the axillary vein, sometimes into the arm, which of course renders any possibility of surgical intervention impossible (Fig. 13.4).

J.E. Molina, *New Techniques for Thoracic Outlet Syndromes*,
DOI 10.1007/978-1-4614-5471-7_13,

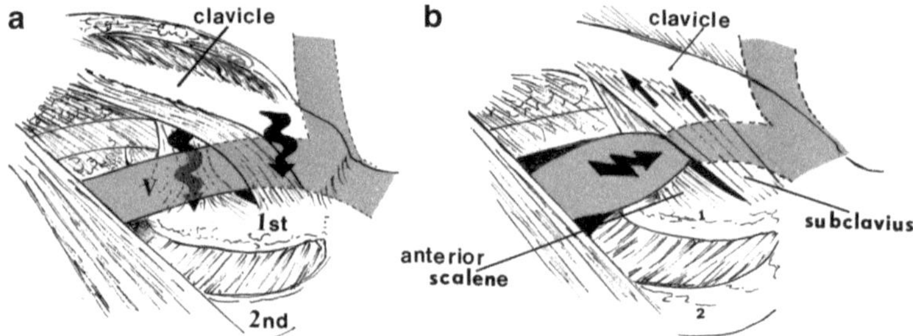

Fig. 13.1 This illustration shows the thoracic inlet tunnel through which the subclavian vein runs into the mediastinum. (**a**) In the relaxed normal position the subclavian vein runs between the subclavius muscle tendon and the anterior scalene muscle. The floor of the tunnel is formed by the 1st rib. (**b**) Under tension the vein is pinched severely between the subclavius tendon and the anterior scalene muscle. Endothelial injury results and evolves into acute thrombosis of the vessel

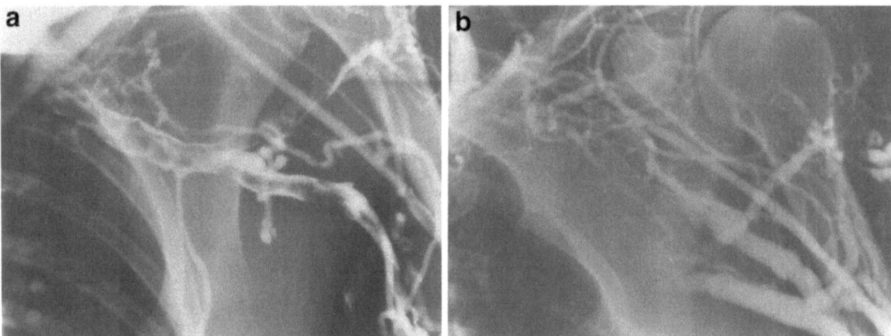

Fig. 13.2 (**a**) Venogram of the left subclavian vein showing total obstruction at the level of the thoracic inlet and multiple thrombus along the axillary and subclavian vein evident by the nonopacification of the vessel. (**b**) Total obstruction of the axillary and subclavian veins prior to implementation of thrombolytic therapy. Reprinted, with permission, from Molina JE et al. Protocols for Paget-Schroetter Syndrome and late treatment of chronic subclavian vein obstruction. *Annals Thoracic Surgery* 2009;87:416–22

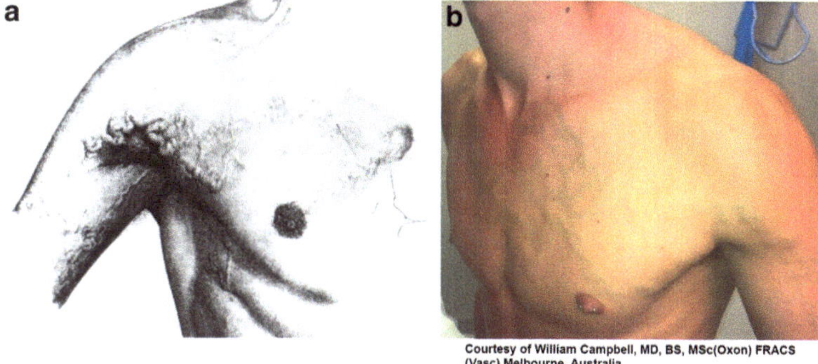

Fig. 13.3 (**a**) This is from the Von Schroetter report. Looking at the illustration of the degree of congestion and tortuosity of the veins, it indicates that the patient had already a chronic obstruction with significant amount of collaterals already formed. (**b**) A 24-year-old man with chronic obstruction of the subclavian vein (Courtesy of William Campbell MD, BS, MSc (Oxon) FRACS (Vasc) Melbourne, Australia)

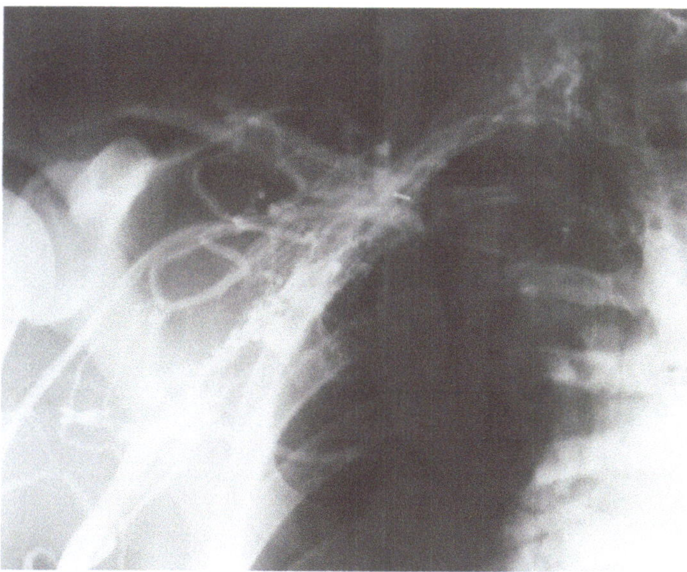

Fig. 13.4 33-year-old woman evaluated 2 months after the original event. Inoperable for reconstruction. Reprinted, with permission, from Molina JE. Need of emergency treatment in subclavian vein effort thrombosis. Journal of American College of Surgeons 1995;181:414–20

Reference

1. Schroetter VL. Erkrankungen der Gefasse. Northnagel Handbuch der Pathologie und Therapie. Wien: Alfred Holder; 1884.

Chapter 14
Venous Obstructions Due to Implanted Devices

Scientific advances over the past 30 years or so have also caused new problems including those caused when devices of several sorts are implanted into the subclavian and less often into the jugular veins [1, 2]. These include insertion of pacemaker leads to treat cardiac arrhythmias, defibrillator leads to treat and prevent sudden death due to ventricular fibrillation, catheters for dialysis [3] when IV fistulas either cannot be used or are being constructed, central venous catheters used for prolonged infusion of antibiotics or chemotherapeutic agents, and central intravenous alimentation lines. Whenever a catheter simply touches venous endothelium fibrotic reaction can occur and in the worst-case scenario may lead to total obliteration of the superior vena cava. These are obviously very complicated and difficult problems to treat, especially when total obstruction of the veins occurs. They may become overwhelming when venous sites of the opposite side are utilized transferring the problem to other veins which will be affected in the same manner.

References

1. Lumsden AB, MacDonald MJ, Isiklar H, et al. Central venous stenosis in the hemodialysis patient: incidence and efficacy of endovascular treatment. Cardiovasc Surg. 1997;5:504–9.
2. Kock HJ, Dietsch M, Kravse U, Wilke H, Eigler FW. Implantable vascular access system: experience in 1500 patients with totally implanted central venous port systems. World J Surg. 1998;22:12–6.
3. Seelig MH, Oldenburg WA, Klinger PJ, Odell JA. Superior vena cava syndrome caused by chronic hemodialysis catheters: autologous reconstruction with a pericardial tube graft. J Vasc Surg. 1998;28:556–60.

J.E. Molina, *New Techniques for Thoracic Outlet Syndromes*,
DOI 10.1007/978-1-4614-5471-7_14,

Chapter 15
Diagnosis

A. Duplex Ultrasound

The first line of approach to make a diagnosis is to use a duplex ultrasound of the axillary subclavian veins. Any patient showing up at the emergency room with a swollen arm should have this test done before assuming any other etiologies that could cause edema of the upper extremity. It is a very simple noninvasive test that will make the diagnosis immediately. There is no need to apply any type of maneuvers implemented on the arm which may actually be contraindicated because if a thrombosis exists abduction of the arm may trigger fragmentation of the clot and cause pulmonary embolism. Typically the tracing will show dampening of the vein pulsations (Fig. 15.1) and total lack of flow which may extend into the axillary vein and occasionally even into the brachial veins. With this information confirmed the next mandatory test is to proceed with a venogram.

B. Venography

This is accomplished by injecting contrast medium in the brachial vein to assess the extent of the thrombosis as well as to assess the severity of the process. Because the arm may be severely edematous and difficult to identify the veins for proper cannulation, an ultrasound can be used to locate the proper vein for an adequate puncture. Occasionally if this is impossible to do other resources are to proceed with a more complicated test like an MRV that may help to determine the degree of thrombosis and its extent. In our experience it is almost never necessary to proceed along these lines and the simple venogram will give much better information and is always feasible to obtain. With this information obtained the next step is to begin the treatment of the process which is described in the following section.

J.E. Molina, *New Techniques for Thoracic Outlet Syndromes*,
DOI 10.1007/978-1-4614-5471-7_15,

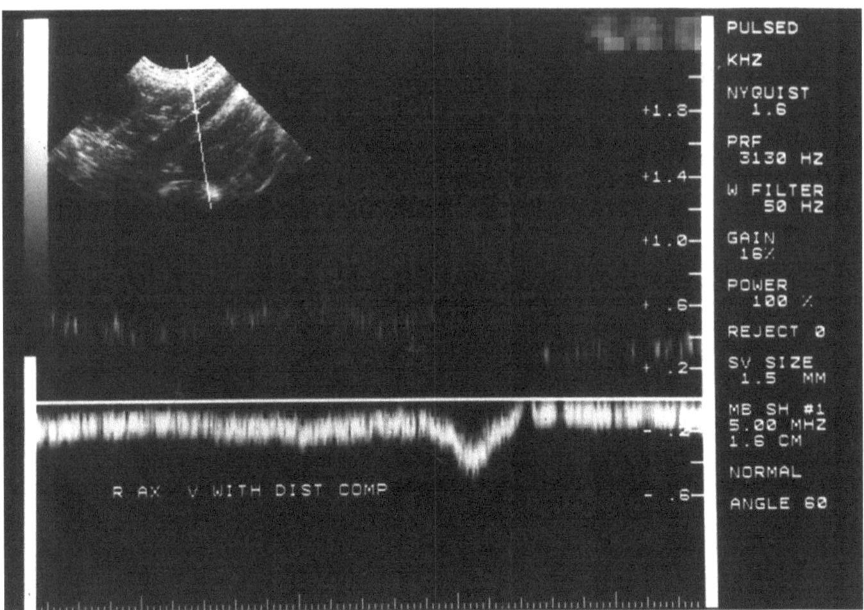

Fig. 15.1 Duplex ultrasound obtained in a patient with acute obstruction of the subclavian vein. The tracing is damped. The only spike seen is upon compressing manually the upper arm

C. Interventional Radiologic Techniques

The radiologist must be able to apply several techniques to help solve the problems associated with the Paget–Schroetter syndrome. In the face of an acute obstruction, it is standard practice, first, to make the diagnosis using a duplex ultrasound exam (Fig. 15.1) after which the radiologist should proceed with a venogram to assess the extent and severity of the obstruction. Next, it is necessary to dissolve the clot using catheter-directed infusion of thrombolytic agents (Fig. 15.2) and occasionally to employ a thrombectomy catheter. We prefer to use thrombolytic agents to gradually dissolve the clot but without causing any trauma to the vein wall proximally or distally. It is an effective and rapid procedure, which usually dissolves the subclavian vein thrombus in less than 24 h (Fig. 15.3a–c). This leaves an open vein with an endothelium which is either intact or only very lightly damaged. This is optimal for the next step: surgery to lay a vein patch to enlarge the diameter of the vein, which has been our preferred approach for the past 20 years [1–4]. On the other hand, use of a thrombectomy catheter initially is quite likely to damage the venous endothelium, particularly if it is attempted more than once. We have observed a number of cases in which “successful” initial thrombectomy leads to reocclusion even in anticoagulated patients. Accordingly surgery should be undertaken immediately after the first clearing. This is true because the radiologist frequently decides on another

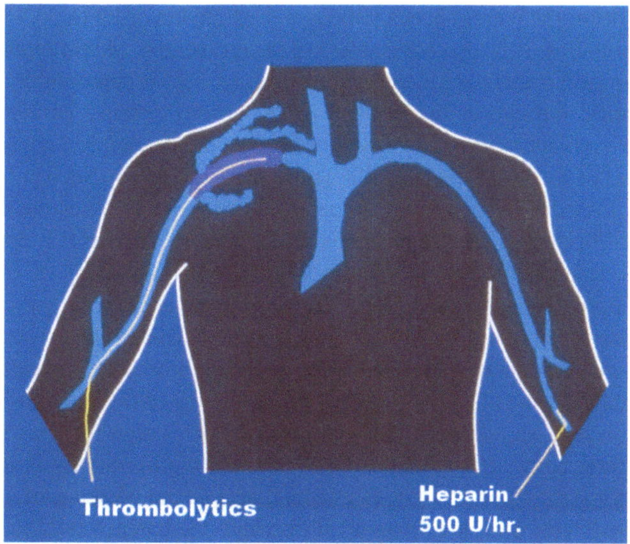

Fig. 15.2 Infusion catheter in position to administer thrombolytics

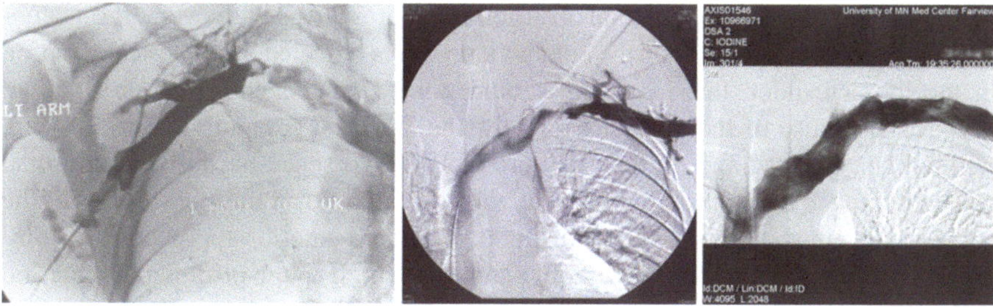

Fig. 15.3 Two examples showing the effect of thrombolytic therapy (Urokinase). (**a**) After 1 h of infusion showing exactly the tight short obstruction of the subclavian vein in the thoracic inlet. (**b**) After 2 h of TNK infusion and (**c**) following surgical repair with vein patch implant and stenting. Reprinted, with permission, from Molina JE et al. Paget-Schroetter Syndrome treated with thrombolytics and immediate surgery. *Journal of Vascular Surgery* 2007;45:328–34

attempt using the thrombectomy catheter to reopen the vein which almost invariably causes more damage to the endothelium. Further, because the extrinsic compression remains unchanged, if no surgery is undertaken, the vein will invariably reocclude. For all these reasons, the ideal time to intervene surgically is immediately after the vein is cleared of fresh clot. Failure to treat patients in this way has resulted in total fibrotic obstruction of not only the subclavian vein but also of the axillary and brachial veins. In this circumstance, surgical intervention of any sort is impossible leaving the patient totally disabled for life with a useless arm (Fig. 13.4).

An additional problem associated with the use of thrombectomy catheters is that destruction of a large thrombus can cause hemoglobinuria of a significant degree.

Should this occur the patient needs to be well hydrated in order to prevent plugging of the renal tubules. It is also advisable to add intravenous Mannitol and diuretics, all in an effort to protect the kidneys from forming tubular hemoglobin plugs.

One specific indication for the use of the thrombectomy catheter is in the postoperative patient who has rethrombosed after the decompressive surgery with the placement of a venous patch to enlarge the subclavian vein. Such patients should undergo an immediate same-day postoperative venogram to asses the status of the repair. If total occlusion with rethrombosis has, in fact, occurred it is appropriate to use thrombectomy catheter to clear the vein before implanting an endovascular stent. This approach has worked well for us because it accelerates patient recovery without exposing the need for thrombolytic therapy, which may cause bleeding in this immediate postoperative period. The use of the thrombectomy catheter in this manner is effective and allows for a total solution to the obstructive problem thanks to the placement of an endovascular stent. A principal reason for insisting on postoperative venography after initial surgery in these circumstances is its ability to detect residual stenosis of the venous channel, despite the presence of a vein patch. It then becomes very simple to pass a catheter into the patent vessel to implant the stent. Fortunately in over 200 cases operated for subclavian vein thrombosis we have had to use this approach only in four cases.

Occasionally patients are encountered who are symptomatic from vein compression even without developing total obstruction or thrombosis of the vein. If on venogram a significant stenosis of the subclavian vein is detected at its typical location in the thoracic inlet, these patients should not be treated with balloon dilation, because the cause of the problem, namely, the extrinsic compression of the vein, will not be corrected and, in fact, will probably be worsened because of additional catheter damage to the endothelium. Patients with significant fibrotic stenosis of the subclavian vein should be operated using the standard anterior approach to decompress the thoracic inlet with or without patch implant. If in the postoperative period the venogram shows residual stenosis an endovascular stent can then easily be implanted.

In summary if a patient has not obstructed the vein totally but is symptomatic with recurring edema of the hand and is found on venography to have stenosis of the subclavian vein, he or she should be operated upon. Attempts to enlarge the diameter of the vein using balloon plasties only lead to more problems and are almost never effective as a permanent solution.

In cases of acute thrombosis (Paget–Schroetter syndrome), catheter-directed infusion of thrombolytic agents to clear the clot until the site of the obstruction can be clearly visualized is completely appropriate if the surgical procedure is then undertaken immediately after the vein is cleared. The use of thrombectomy catheters should be reserved for the circumstance when a postoperative venogram following vein patch plasty shows rethrombosis. In such a case, the clot should be removed with the catheter and endovascular stent can be implanted simultaneously without exposing the patient to further use of thrombolytic agents.

The implant of endovascular stents is usually required in cases with chronic obstruction and is only needed in about 10 % of the cases with acute obstruction, because the vein patch angioplasty is usually sufficient to restore the normal caliber of the subclavian vein. However, in chronic cases significant amount of venous fibrosis exists so that, even when the thoracic inlet is decompressed and the vein is patched, the vein walls are so fibrosed that they have the tendency to collapse again. If this is apparent on postoperative venogram, the use of a stent is usually mandatory. The diameter size of the stent to be implanted varies upon the size of the patient, but usually in an adult a size 10–14 mm in diameter is usually effective and restores the normal flow in the subclavian vein.

References

1. Molina JE. Surgery for effort thrombosis of the subclavian vein. J Thorac Cardiovasc Surg. 1992;103:341–6.
2. Molina JE. Treatment of chronic obstruction of the axillary, subclavian, and innominate veins. Int J Angiol. 1999;8:87–90.
3. Molina JE, Hunter DW, Dietz CA. Paget-Schroetter syndrome treated with thrombolytics and immediate surgery. J Vasc Surg. 2007;45:328–34.
4. Molina JE, Hunter DW, Dietz CA. Protocols for Paget-Schroetter syndrome and late treatment of chronic subclavian vein obstruction. Ann Thorac Surg. 2009;87:416–22.

Chapter 16
The New Treatment Approach to Subclavian Vein Thrombosis

The first step in treating Paget–Schroetter syndrome is to initiate anticoagulation in order to prevent further thrombus formation, and propagation into the distal arm as well as to prevent pulmonary thromboembolism. Once the diagnosis is made the patient should be placed on intravenous heparin peripherally using a high intensity regimen: a bolus of 100 u/kg intravenously in a vein of the non-affected arm, followed by continuous intravenous infusion at a rate preferably determined by monitoring the Xa which must reach a level of 0.3–0.7 to be effective. If the medical center is still using the PTT methodology (partial thromboplastin time) this should reach levels between 60 and 80. Before initiating heparin therapy platelet count must be obtained and monitored to detect the development of heparin Induced Thrombocytopenia (HIT). The platelet count can drop drastically and rapidly if patients develop this syndrome. If this complication occurs, heparin must be immediately discontinued and a different anticoagulant employed.

Heparin alone will not solve the problem, however, and should only be considered as a temporary adjuvant to more definitive therapy. The preferable next step is to implement thrombolytic therapy for rapid resolution of the process. If the medical center in which the patient is seen initially does not have the ability to carry out thrombolytic therapy, the patient should be transferred immediately to one that does. The patient should always be transferred with intravenous heparin running to arrest the thrombotic process. This is only a temporary measure until full anticoagulation is established and a therapeutic plan is established to achieve prolonged anticoagulation. In Paget–Schroetter syndrome Lovenox (low weight heparin) should be only used temporarily especially postoperatively until an adequate level of anticoagulation can be achieved using warfarin. Also of importance: when intravenous heparin is used, only porcine mucosal heparin is indicated rather than the beef lung heparin commonly used in the past, because it is less likely to cause HIT syndromes, and/or allergic reactions. The porcine mucosa heparin is prescribed as units per kilogram patient weight, and not in milligrams as is the case for beef lung heparin. If the patient is known to be sensitive to the heparin or has developed HIT in the past, a different anticoagulant like argatroban or hirudin should be chosen.

J.E. Molina, *New Techniques for Thoracic Outlet Syndromes*,
DOI 10.1007/978-1-4614-5471-7_16,

Unfortunately, both are harder to monitor and have a higher risk for bleeding elsewhere. Therefore, their administration must be properly and closely monitored.

Although anticoagulants are routinely used after many types of vascular surgery, they are especially indicated in venous surgery because veins are more prone to thrombosis due to the low pressure system, easily collapsible vein walls, and are subject to intermittent stasis all of which leads to thrombosis, particularly after operations for Paget–Schroetter syndrome which involve placement of vein patch with or without placement of endovascular stents. Our preference is for Coumadin (warfarin), clopidogrel (Plavix), Dextran (Rheomacrodex 40), Lovenox (low weight heparin) as further explained in this section.

Chapter 17
Timing for Intervention and Standard of Care

From its initial reports it was clear that prompt intervention was indicated to treat subclavian vein thrombosis. In an extensive review published in 1934 [1] Matas, recognized that, even though etiology of the problem was unknown at that time, the presence of persistent edema and pain in the arm warranted an urgent exploratory operation. He recommended thrombectomy, because, in his words, "waiting was not a logical option; so called expectant treatment should yield without too a long delay to surgical exploration for the seat of the lesion." Läwen [2] in 1937 proposed the same approach and reported several cases of thrombectomy, noting that the earlier the thrombectomy was undertaken, the better the results obtained in relieving the symptoms of venous obstruction. Drapanas [3] reported a small series of cases treated with emergency thrombectomy with good reestablishment of flow and gratifying relief of symptoms. He stressed that emergency thrombectomy appeared to offer the best possibility for restoring the upper extremity to normal in a very short period of time using a relatively simple procedure and to prevent extensive organization of thrombus, therefore avoiding all sequels of this disease. Mahorner and others came to believe [4] that removal of the thrombus in the early stage was the only procedure of any benefit to treat this condition.

Aziz and colleagues [5] stated clearly the two aims of early intervention: removal of the obstructing thrombus and correction of the constrictive mechanism extrinsic to the vein at the thoracic inlet. Based on these considerations, urgent decompression of the thoracic inlet, dissolution of the thrombus and reestablishment of the normal caliber of the subclavian vein at the thoracic inlet is the policy at the University of Minnesota [6–8]. The acute venous thrombosis of the axillary subclavian complex is treated immediately with thrombolytic agents in order to visualize the anatomy of the vein and to evaluate the degree and extent of the obstruction. All of this is necessary in order to plan a proper operation. We were among the first to point out the need for emergency treatment of the subclavian vein effort thrombosis in 1995 [8]. A year later, Rutherford and Hulburt [9] explored the experience of a panel of 25 expert vascular surgeons with the problem and found that 70% of them were of the opinion that thrombectomy should be performed within 5 days to obtain a reasonable chance of success. They also thought that the 10 day waiting limit was

J.E. Molina, *New Techniques for Thoracic Outlet Syndromes*,
DOI 10.1007/978-1-4614-5471-7_17,

Table 17.1 Subclavian vein "effort" thrombosis

Evolution without emergency lytic therapy and surgery
1. Total obliteration occurs rapidly
2. Vein fibrosis extends into arm veins and innominate
3. Possibility to reestablish patency is diminished or lost >2 weeks
4. Irreversible chronic arm edema and pain
5. Permanent disability to use the arm

still reasonable, but longer periods of delay had much less chance of success in reestablishing the proper venous channel. Zimmerman et al. [10] found residual thrombus in 100% of patients treated beyond 10 days compared to 14% in those treated before 10 days from the original event. Similar results were reported by Wilson [11]: residual clot was found in 100% of patients treated 7 days after the event versus only 29% in those treated before 7 days. Therefore, the general current opinion is that treatment with thrombolytic agents should be implemented in less than 14 days after the onset (Table 17.1). In fact, a large majority of surgeons favored the operation without waiting for residual symptoms to reappear which occur almost all within 3–4 weeks of the event or during the same hospitalization. There seems little doubt therefore that the standard of care in treating subclavian vein thrombosis entails the prompt initial use of thrombolytic agents followed immediately by surgery as indicated by us in several publications [12–17].

References

1. Matas R. On the so-called primary thrombosis of the axillary vein caused by strain. Am J Surg. 1934;24:642–66.
2. Läwen VA. Über thrombektomie bei venenthrombose und arteriospasmus. Zentrblatt chirurg. 1937;17:961–8.
3. Drapanas T, Curran WL. Thrombectomy in the treatment of "effort" thrombosis of the axillary and subclavian veins. J Trauma. 1966;6:107–19.
4. Mahorner H, Castleberry JW, Coleman WO. Attempts to restore function in major veins which are the site of massive thrombosis. Ann Surg. 1957;146:510–22.
5. Aziz S, Straehley CJ, Wheland Jr TJ. Effort-related axillosubclavian vein thrombosis. A new theory of pathogenesis and a plea for direct surgical intervention. Am J Surg. 1986;152: 57–61.
6. Molina JE, Hunter DW, Dietz CA. Paget-Schroetter syndrome treated with thrombolytics and immediate surgery. J Vasc Surg. 2007;45:328–34.
7. Molina JE, Hunter DW, Dietz CA. Protocols for Paget-Schroetter syndrome and late treatment of chronic subclavian vein obstruction. Ann Thorac Surg. 2009;87:416–22.
8. Molina JE. Need for emergency treatment in subclavian vein effort thrombosis. J Am Coll Surg. 1995;181:414–20.
9. Rutherford RB, Hurlbert SN. Primary subclavian-axillary vein thrombosis: consensus and commentary. Cardiovasc Surg. 1996;4:420–3.
10. Zimmerman R, Morl H, Harenberg J, et al. Urokinase therapy of subclavian-axillary vein thrombosis. Klin Wochenschr. 1981;59:851–6.

11. Wilson JJ, Zahn CA, Newman H. Fibrinolytic therapy for idiopathic subclavian-axillary vein thrombosis. Am J Surg. 1990;159:208–11.
12. Adams JT, DeWeese JA. "Effort" thrombosis of the axillary and subclavian veins. J Trauma. 1971;11:923–30.
13. DeLeon RA, Chang DC, Hassown H, Black JH, Roseborough GS, et al. Multiple treatment algorithms for successful ouitcomes in venous throracic outlet syndromes. Surgery. 2009; 145:500–7.
14. Azakie A, McElhinney DB, Thompson RW, et al. Surgical management of subclavian-vein effort thrombosis as a result of thoracic outlet compression. J Vasc Surg. 1998;28:777–86.
15. Swinton Jr NW, Edgett JW, Hall RJ. Primary subclavian-axillary vein thrombosis. Circulation. 1968;38:737–45.
16. Landercasper J, Gall W, Fisher M, et al. Thrombolytic therapy of axillary-subclavian venous thrombosis. Arch Surg. 1987;122:1072–5.
17. Urschel Jr HC, Razzuk MA. Paget-Schroetter syndrome: what is the best management? Ann Thorac Surg. 2000;69:1663–9.

Chapter 18
Thrombolytic Therapy

As already noted, catheter directed infusion of thrombolytics is very effective in dissolving the clot within a short period of time, usually less than 24 h [1–3]. Once the thrombus is dissolved then the surgeon can use venography to assess the severity of the obstruction and its length, critical parameters to evaluate and plan for the next stage. In our institution, the thrombolytic agent of choice was until 1999 Urokinase when it was removed from the market. Since then RTPA products have been used, primarily Tenecteplase (TNK; Genentech, South San Francisco, CA); and Alteplase (Activase, Genentech) both delivered at the dose of 0.05 mg/kg/h, (average 0.25 mg/h) (Table 18.1). Tenecteplase has been both effective and safe in our hands during the past 11 years. In addition, it is the least expensive. Most of interventional radiologists are familiar with both drugs which, when administered at the doses indicated are very safe and almost free of complications. The only important monitoring test during the thrombolytic infusion is the fibrinogen level. Because of the thrombotic process, all these patients demonstrate high levels of fibrinogen when they arrive at the hospital. Deviations from the normal level of fibrinogen found in blood (300 mg%) values as high as 700–800 mg% are not uncommon. Once the infusion of thrombolytic agents is underway, these levels tend to drop. Further, in the short period of 24 h required fibrinogen levels rarely drop to levels less than 150 mg%, the lower limit required to prevent bleeding. We currently do not measure fibrinogen split products or other more complicated tests, because these results cannot be reported to the treating physician within 30 min of drawing the blood, not the case with the fibrinogen levels.

After initiating thrombolytic therapy, the venogram should be repeated 8–12 h later to assess the need for further infusion or for reposition of the catheter in areas that have not been cleared. If the infusion of thrombolytic agents is prolonged beyond 24 h, it is important to monitor the fibrinogen level frequently. If it falls to

J.E. Molina, *New Techniques for Thoracic Outlet Syndromes*,
DOI 10.1007/978-1-4614-5471-7_18,

Table 18.1 Thrombolytic dosage direct infusion

Agent	Hourly	Avg.	Adjusted
TNK	0.25–0.3 mg/h	0.25	0.05 mg/kg/h
Alteplase	0.2–10 mg/h	0.35	0.05 mg/kg/h
Reteplase	0.5–1.0 U/h	0.75	0.01 U/kg/h
Urokinase	150,000 U/h	150,000	2,200 U/kg/h

the 150 mg% or less infusion is stopped until the fibrinogen levels return to a higher level. After 24 h, any remaining thrombus-like formation in the vein represents chronic organized fibrotic thrombosis which will have to be removed surgically. There is no justification for prolonging the thrombolytic infusion. At this point, the patient is taken to the operating room to repair the vein and to decompress the thoracic inlet. Because thrombolytic therapy has become such a mainstay in the treatment of Paget–Schroetter syndrome, close cooperation and coordination between the interventional radiologist and the surgeon is mandatory.

During the period of thrombolytic infusion, intravenous heparin should be administered in the contralateral arm at a rate of 500 units/h. As soon as complete dissolution of the clot is achieved, thrombolytic infusion is discontinued and the heparin infusion is increased to 1,000 units/h until the time of surgery. Other coagulation parameters must also be checked preoperatively (INR, PTT, platelet count, and thrombin time), because they will be useful in directing anticoagulation therapy in the postoperative period. It should be emphasized that heparin is discontinued approximately 2 h before beginning the next step, the operative procedure.

Frequentlly, if a patient is seen longer than 2 weeks from the original event, organized thrombus may well be present which cannot be dissolved. In these cases, the thrombus must be removed under direct vision at the time of surgery. Even though the thrombolytic therapy has been terminated and the catheter removed, the infusion sheath, however, should be left in place, because this will be used immediately after surgery to perform a post operative venogram and verify the effectiveness of the venous repair, assessment of whether or not the patch placed on the stenotic segment of the vein is optimal or whether or not residual stenosis still persists. In that case the radiologist using the same sheath can introduce catheters to do balloon angioplasty with placement of stents.

With the new research being done on the use of new and safer thrombolytic agents some of them have shown already in clinical trials to be more effective and less risky than the current ones. One of them is the Desmoteplase [4], which is a novel highly fibrin specific thrombolytic agent at the present time in Phase III of clinical development. Its structure is similar to rTPA (Alteplase), but it does not contain the plasmin-sensitive cleavage site and as a result this multiplase in comparison with rTPA has fibrin selectivity, absence of neurotoxicity and apparently no negative effects on the blood–brain barrier. So far we have not used this agent neither is it approved for treatment of peripheral venous thrombosis. Nevertheless we should keep in mind that new discoveries are being made continuously and we should be alert to implement whatever is safer to take care of our patients.

References

1. Molina JE, Hunter DW, Dietz CA. Paget-Schroetter syndrome treated with thrombolytics and immediate surgery. J Vasc Surg. 2007;45:328–34.
2. Zimmerman R, Morl H, Harenberg J, et al. Urokinase therapy of subclavian-axillary vein thrombosis. Klin Wochenschr. 1981;59:851–6.
3. Wilson JJ, Zahn CA, Newman H. Fibrinolytic therapy for idiopathic subclavian-axillary vein thrombosis. Am J Surg. 1990;159:208–11.
4. Schleuning WD. Vampire bat plasminogen activator DSPA-alpha-1 (desmoteplase): a thrombolytic drug optimized by natural selection. Hemostasis. 2001;31(3–6):118–22.

Chapter 19
Surgical Intervention

The New Subclavicular Approach Operation

An incision is made parallel to the clavicle approximately 1–1½ in. below this level. The incision should extend from the lateral border of the sternum towards the delto-pectoral groove (Fig. 19.1). After entering the subcutaneous tissue, the fibers of the pectoralis major are encountered. Usually a groove or natural separation of the fibers of the pectoralis major muscle exists, one group going to the clavicle and the other group towards the sternum. The incision is continued in that groove by splitting the muscle fibers bluntly without cutting or dividing them. This allows the surgeon to reach the retropectoral space exactly on top of the first rib. The adipose tissue is dissected and reflected laterally in order to expose the rib cage (Fig. 19.2). In severe cases of venous obstruction, it is necessary to inspect for the presence of dilated lymphatic channels which may be seen reaching the subclavian vein. These must be divided and tied securely in order to prevent post operative lymphatic drainage.

After clearing this area, the first rib is visualized and the subclavius tendon, first structure encountered towards the middle of the incision is identified (Fig. 19.3). This is easily dissected using the cautery, separating it from the fibers of the pectoralis major muscle superiorly. As its lateral border it must be separated and dissected off the anterior surface of the subclavian vein immediately underneath (Fig. 19.4).

Once this is accomplished, the insertion of the tendon on the first rib is divided using the cautery. Usually an Allis forceps can be applied to the cut end of the tendon and deflected upwards in order to continue detachment of the muscle off the clavicle and the subclavian vein (Fig. 19.5a, b). The muscle is detached from the under surface of the clavicle and further reflected up and more laterally until it is completely freed from the surrounding structures for a distance of at least 1½–2 in. At this level, muscle is divided and removed from the field. The costoclavicular ligament is immediately underneath and is also divided and resected. Often, the surgeon at this point falls into the capsule of the costoclavicular joint, but this does not interfere with any part of the operation and does not cause any damage to the function of this joint. Attention is directed towards the subclavian vein, which is now fully visualized

J.E. Molina, *New Techniques for Thoracic Outlet Syndromes*,
DOI 10.1007/978-1-4614-5471-7_19,

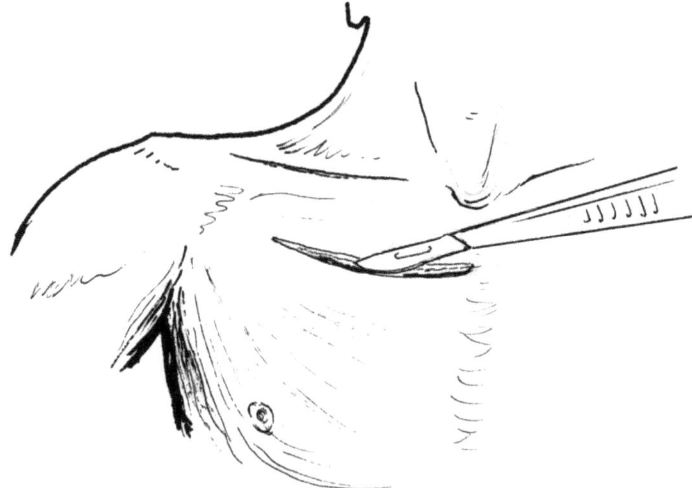

Fig. 19.1 A standard subclavicular incision to approach the subclavian vein in cases of Paget–Schroetter syndrome and chronic obstruction of the subclavian vein. Reprinted, with permission, from Molina JE. Approach to the confluence of the subclavian and internal jugular veins without claviculectomy. *Seminars in Vascular Surgery* 2000;13:10–19

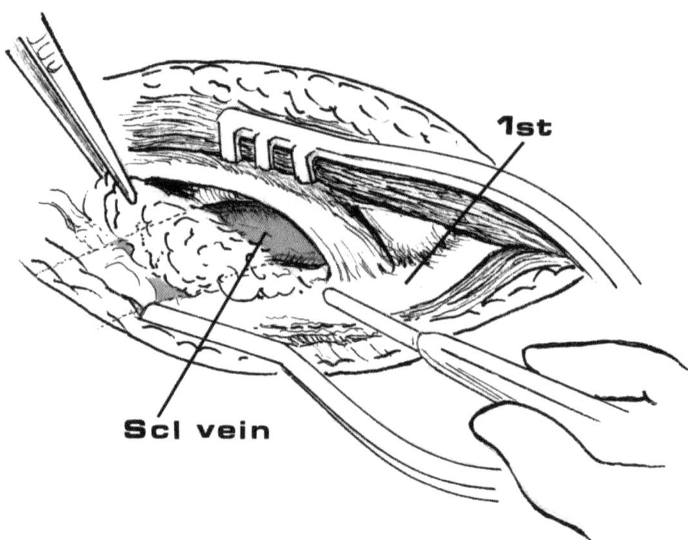

Fig. 19.2 As soon as the pectoralis major muscle is entered by separating its fibers the first structure in front is constituted by the subclavius tendon that crosses anteriorly the subclavian vein. Reprinted, with permission, from Molina JE. Approach to the confluence of the subclavian and internal jugular veins without claviculectomy. *Seminars in Vascular Surgery* 2000;13:10–19

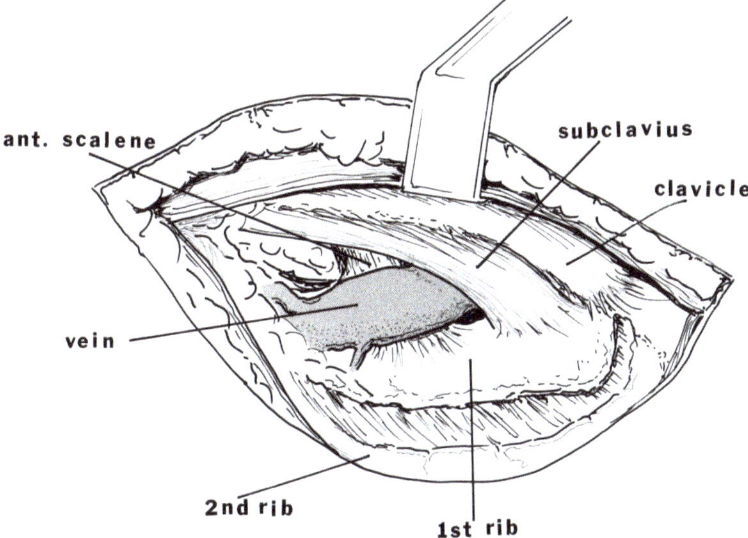

Fig. 19.3 This illustration shows the position of the different structures in the thoracic inlet in their normal relationship as shown by the intraoperative photograph

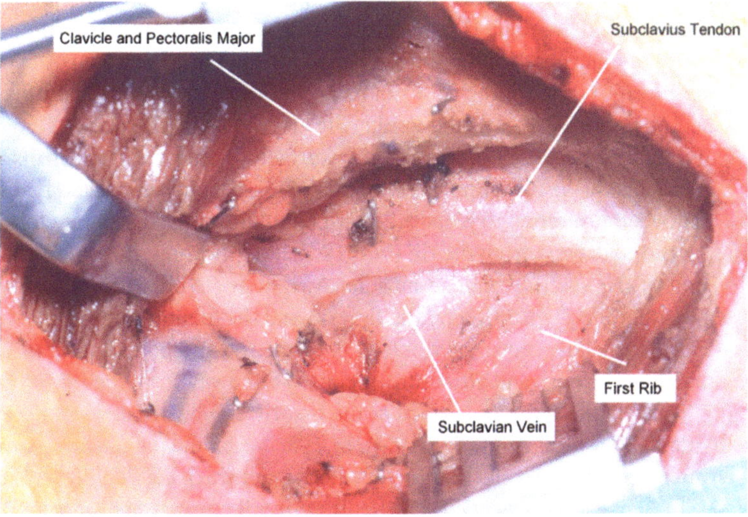

Fig. 19.4 Intraoperative photograph of a patient with right subclavian vein thrombosis after the pectoralis major muscle has been entered. The subclavian vein is severely compressed between the tendon of the subclavius muscle and the first rib

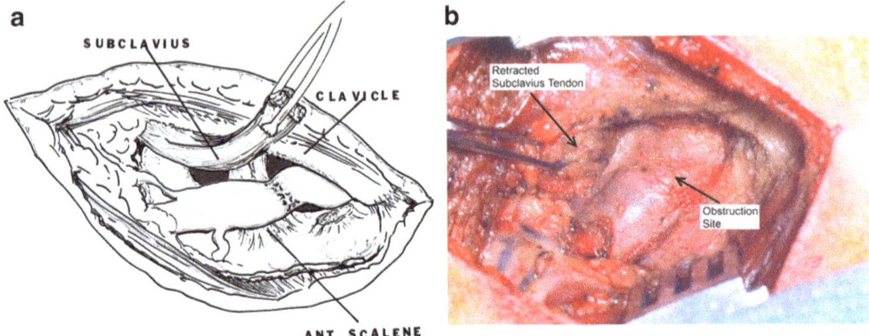

Fig. 19.5 (**a**) The subclavius tendon has been divided at the point of insertion in the first rib and reflected upwards. Immediately it shows the subclavian vein underneath and the level of the constriction in front of the anterior scalene muscle. (**b**) The same patient shown here after the subclavius muscle has been divided and retracted laterally. The site of the obstruction (*arrow*) shows the thickening and indentation of the vein

laying over the superior surface of the first rib. The vein is detached from the rib using the cautery. As the upper border of the vein is dissected off the connective tissue, venous branches coming down from the neck are often encountered. These branches should not be tied off; they do not interfere, and will be controlled with the vascular clamps used at the time the vein is directly repaired. The vein is now freely separated from the first rib and the dissection can proceeds laterally and posteriorly. I usually do not divide the anterior scalene muscle at this point in order to prevent any possibility of entering the pleura. Instead, an incision is now made in the periosteum of the inferior border of the rib from its point of insertion at the sternum going laterally and posteriorly towards the axilla (Fig. 19.6). Using the periosteum elevators, this is then detached from the inferior surface of first rib through its entire length. As soon as this is accomplished, an extra-pleural space is created behind the rib which allows the surgeon to place a finger behind the rib and separate the pleura and the endothoracic facia from the rib (Fig. 19.7). At this point, it is safe to proceed with division of the anterior scalene muscle. A right angle clamp is placed around the base of its tendinous insertion on the first rib and the tendon is divided using the cautery (Fig. 19.8). This sequence of steps prevents the surgeon from accidentally entering the pleural cavity and allows the pleura to fall away from the rib so that any remaining fibers on the superior surface of the first rib can be divided safely. The rib is now divided at its sternal end (Fig. 19.9). In cases when the patient is so muscular that, even after separating the pleura from the inferior surface of the first rib, the surgeon cannot see the anterior scalene muscle, I often divide the rib first at the point of attachment to the sternum. By pressing the mobile rib down against the chest cavity, the anterior scalene muscle tendon is easily exposed. In any case, while dividing the anterior scalene muscle either before or after transecting the rib, the subclavian vein must be held upwards away from the rib using a Langenbeck retractor. This maneuver not only protects the vein but also the subclavian artery sitting behind the anterior scalene muscle.

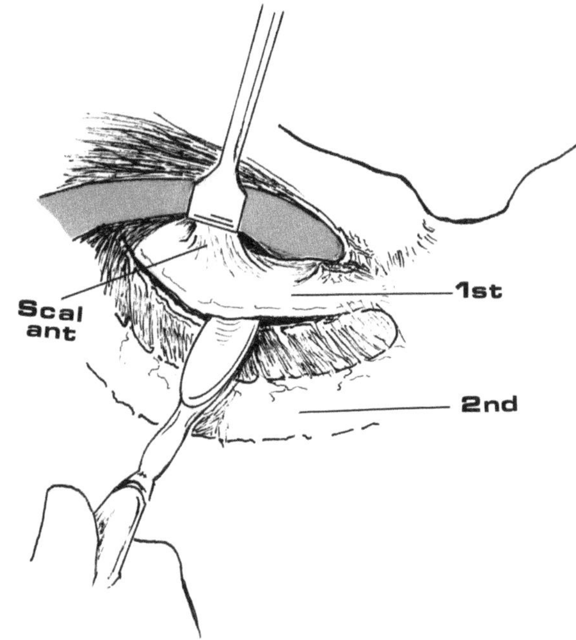

Fig. 19.6 Superiostal dissection of the inferior surface of the first rib in order to create an extrapleural space freeing up the entire rib before the anterior scalene tendon is divided. Reprinted, with permission, from Molina JE. Approach to the confluence of the subclavian and internal jugular veins without claviculectomy. *Seminars in Vascular Surgery* 2000;13:10–19

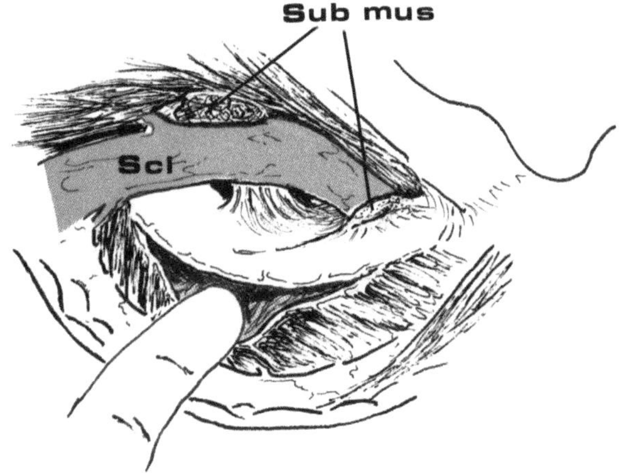

Fig. 19.7 The subclavius muscle has been resected exposing the subclavian vein in front of the anterior scalene muscle. The inferior surface of the first rib has been dissected superiostically until a finger can be passed in the extrapleural space before approaching the anterior scalene muscle for its division

The rib is now completely isolated. Retracting the vein superiorly at the lateral end of the incision the rib is now divided at this level using either a Roos rib cutter or a similar instrument (Fig. 19.10). The segment of rib is removed from the field, and the remaining posterior end of the rib is checked for potential periosteum bleeders which are controlled with the cautery. The next step, which is the most important one to assure success of the operation, is the mobilization of the subclavian vein

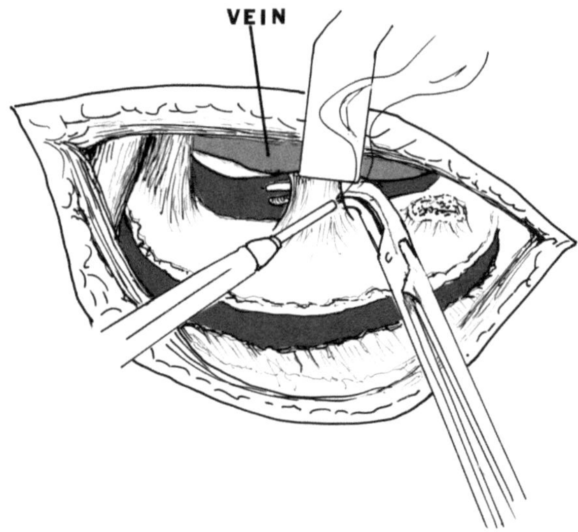

Fig. 19.8 After the extrapleural space is created by superiostal dissection of the first rib then it is safe to pass a right angle forceps around the anterior scalene muscle tendon which is divided using the cautery. At this point it is perfectly safe and this sequence avoids the occurrence of pneumothorax

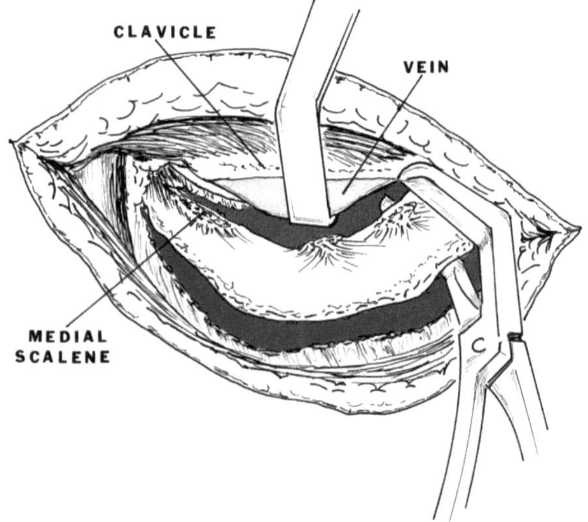

Fig. 19.9 Once the extrapleural space is created by blunt dissection the anterior end of the rib is divided at the level of its insertion in the sternum. The medial scalene muscle is divided as far back as feasible without endangering the nerve roots or the subclavian artery

away from the posterior surface of the manubrium of the sternum [1, 2] (Fig. 19.11). This is done using the cautery while exerting traction on the vein until normal vein is adequately reached beyond the strictured portion. The only branch found in this maneuver is the internal mammary vein running parallel to the lateral border of the sternum. This vessel does not need to be divided. As, the surgeon continues to detach the vein from the posterior surface of the sternum, the proximal portion of the innominate vein is visualized. This should be palpated and seen clearly to ensure that the vein is normal prior to applying the vascular clamps because it assures that any future patch laid over the strictured portion of the vein can be extended up to

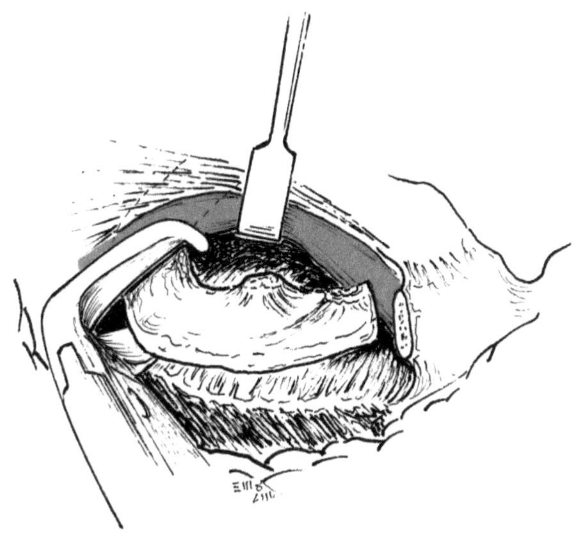

Fig. 19.10 After the anterior scalene muscle is divided and the rib previously transected at its sternal insertion, its posterior end is divided approximately at the level where the subclavian artery crosses the rib. Reprinted, with permission, from Molina JE. Approach to the confluence of the subclavian and internal jugular veins without claviculectomy. *Seminars in Vascular Surgery* 2000;13:10–19

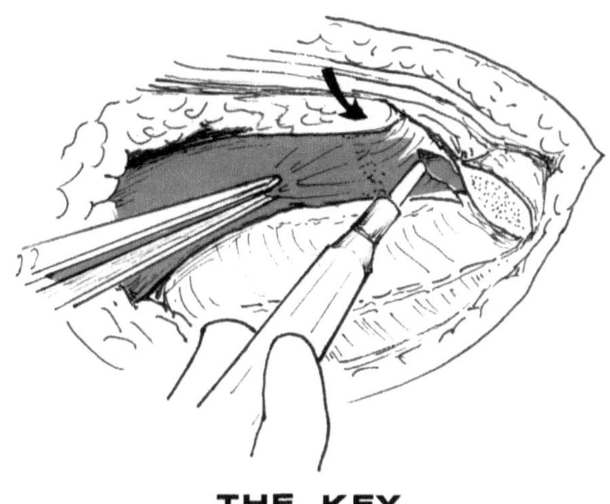

Fig. 19.11 Mobilization of the subclavian vein, detaching it anteriorly from the sternum allowing sufficient margin for placement of the medial clamp. This is the key of success, to lay the future vein patch appropriately. Reprinted, with permission, from Molina JE et al. Paget–Schroetter Syndrome treated with thrombolytics and immediate surgery. *Journal of Vascular Surgery* 2007;45:328–34

normal vein. Note that many of the residual fibers and connective tissue covering the vein at that level can be easily detached using a fine right angle forceps, and cut using the cautery.

Once the medial portion of the dissection is completed, attention is directed to the axillary end of the vein. Most of the time, branches entering the axillary vein can be preserved, but the critical end point of this portion of the operation is to reach a normal portion of the vein, i.e., thin walled and palpable, because it is here that the distal vascular clamp is going to be applied prior to opening the thickened, obstructed portion of the subclavian vein. The operative area is now irrigated many times with antibiotic solution to prevent infection. It should also be completely dry before advancing to the next critical stage: opening the subclavian vein and laying on a patch to widen its diameter. The patient is now given heparin intravenously at the dose of 100 units per kilogram body weight prior to applying the vascular clamp to the vein. Also at this time I usually begin an intravenous infusion of Rheomacrodex (low molecular weight Dextran 40 in 10% dextrose or saline solution) The best way to accomplish this in an adult individual, is to give a bolus of 50 ml over a few minutes followed by a drip at 15 cc per hour. This should be continued postoperatively for 48 h until the level of anticoagulation reaches the therapeutic level induced by the administration of warfarin started the day of surgery. Once the subclavian vein is totally exposed and isolated, attention is directed to the left upper thigh of the patient where a short piece of saphenous vein (usually no more than 6–7 cm) is excised. We use the upper thigh, because the diameter of the saphenous vein at that level is the best for creating an adequately sized vein patch. The vein is excised and distended with heparinized saline and saved for later implantation. The subclavian vein is now clamped I believe it is best to use a spoon shaped Potts vascular clamp on the axillary end of the vein because its curved shape encompasses most of the branches coming down from the neck and upper shoulder. A second clamp to be used has been especially crafted to be applied to the subclavian as it becomes the innominate (Fig. 19.12). It was designed specifically for this operation in order, first, to allow the positioning of its handle to lay flat on the sternum while the vascular anastomosis is undertaken; secondly, the curvature of the clamp usually occludes the external jugular vein coming from the neck, creating a dry field at the time the venotomy is carried out. The vein is now opened lengthwise throughout its entire length (Fig. 19.13a, b). If any residual organized thrombus is present, it is removed. Intermittent release of the clamp on the axillary end of the vein flushes out any residual clots. The site of the obstruction of the vein is now clearly visualized. The vein is usually very thick and has multiple synechia, all of which must be divided and excised. If there is any residual well organized thrombus exists in the area, it must be removed leaving the inner surface of the vein as clean as possible (Fig. 19.14a, b). The saphenous vein segment excised from the thigh is now split lengthwise, tailored properly and then layed over the opening of the vein to widen the stenotic area. The patch is sewn in place with a running 6-0 prolene (Fig. 19.15a–c). Before completion, the clamps are briefly released to flush any residual air and the repair is completed. The entire surgical area is again inspected carefully for potential bleeders, best controlled with the use of the cautery. A soft drain, usually a round Jackson-Pratt, or a size 19 Blake type drain is positioned over the dome of the pleura and brought out through a separate incision on the lateral wall of the chest then connected to bulb suction system to drain any accumulation of fluid. The incision is closed in the usual manner. It is my custom to use nonabsorbable material to approximate the fibers of the pectoralis major, and 3-0 absorbable Vicryl suture to approximate subcutaneous intradermic or subdermic layers. The skin is then sealed with Dermabond. The incision in the thigh is closed in the usual manner using 2-0 or 3-0 Vicryl suture. The patient leaves the operating room without neutralizing the heparin given at the time of the vein clamping, but with the dextran running at 15 cc per hour.

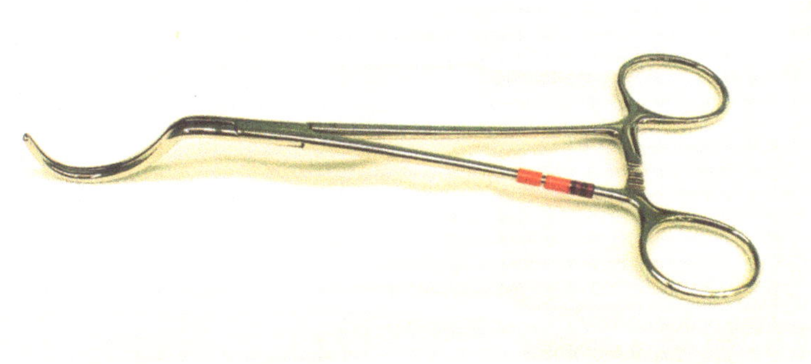

Fig. 19.12 Subclavian vein clamp 2222-167 (Scanlan Instruments. One Scanlan Plaza—St Paul, MN 55107)

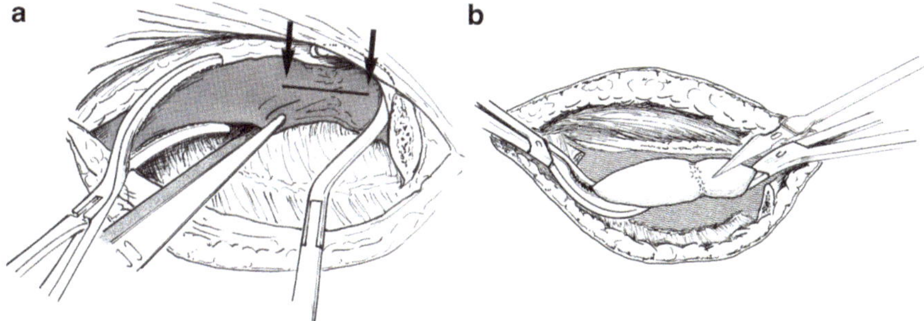

Fig. 19.13 (**a**) The subclavian vein has been clamped at both ends and (**b**) using an 11 bladed knife the vein is opened cutting across the site of the obstruction

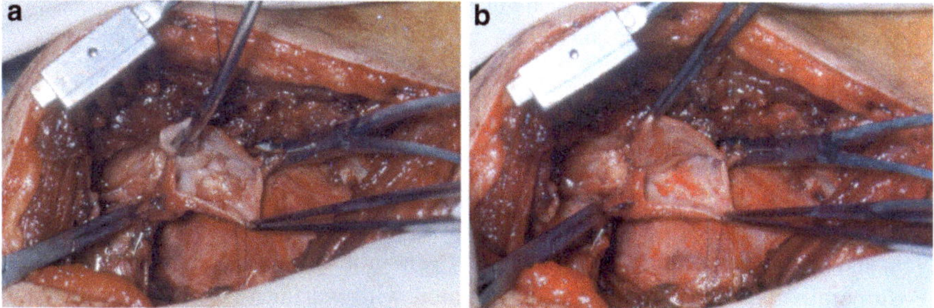

Fig. 19.14 (**a**) The subclavian vein has been opened lengthwise and the lumen is occupied by organized thrombus occluding the lumen at the site of the obstruction. (**b**) After removal of the obstructing materials. Reprinted, with permission, from Molina JE et al. Paget–Schroetter Syndrome treated with thrombolytics and immediate surgery. *Journal of Vascular Surgery* 2007;45:328–34

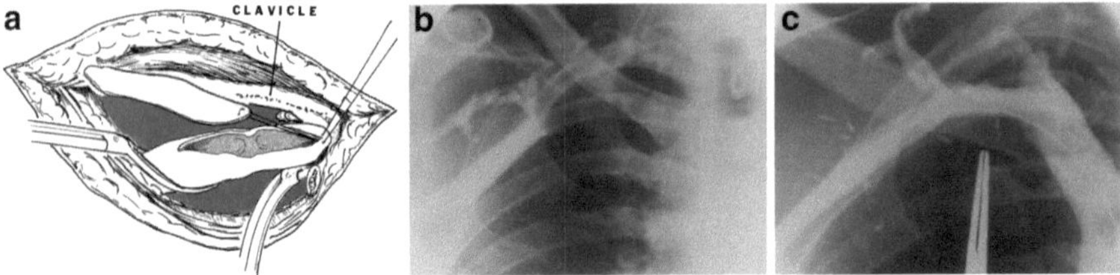

Fig. 19.15 (**a**) After all the synechia and organized fibrous thrombus have been removed from the lumen of the subclavian vein, the saphenous vein patch is now brought into the field and laid over this opening to widen the diameter of the subclavian vein. (**b**) Typical finding of total obstruction of the Subclavian vein at the time of the original thrombotic event. (**c**) After undergoing our standard treatment of thrombolysis and surgical vein patch plasty with decompression of the thoracic inlet. Reprinted, with permission, from Molina JE. Need of emergency treatment in subclavian vein effort thrombosis. *Journal of American College of Surgeons* 1995;181:414–420

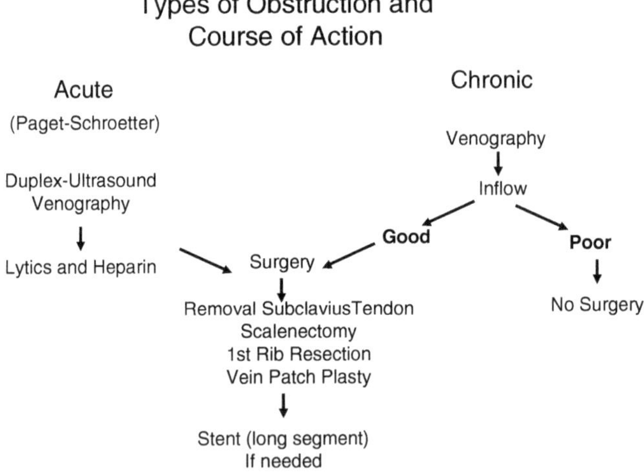

Fig. 19.16 Types of obstruction and course of action

Following our protocol, the patient is now taken to the interventional radiology suite for a post operative venogram to assess the repair. If an area of residual stenosis persists, often the case in cases with chronic fibrous obstruction, the interventional radiologist dilates that portion and inserts a stent to give the vein adequate diameter usually from (10–14 mm in diameter). Once we assess the patency of the vein and detect the presence of good flow by venography the procedure is terminated. Postoperatively, the patient is anticoagulated with warfarin (Coumadin) to reach therapeutic level of INR 2–3 before being discharged home.

The outline of the proper course of action to treat the subclavian vein thrombosis at various stages is displayed on Fig. 19.16. The result of treating this syndrome on emergency basis has rendered a 100 % patency rate (11, 12). This policy will prevent the progression to a chronic inoperable incurable problem leading to permanent arm disability.

References

1. Molina JE, Hunter DW, Dietz CA. Paget-Schroetter syndrome treated with thrombolytics and immediate surgery. J Vasc Surg. 2007;45:328–34.
2. Molina JE, Hunter DW, Dietz CA. Protocols for Paget-Schroetter syndrome and late treatment of chronic subclavian vein obstruction. Ann Thorac Surg. 2009;87:416–22.

Chapter 20
The Transsternal Extension

In some cases, the chronic obstructive fibrotic process involving the subclavian vein extends far medially. In this instance, the standard incision is inadequate to expose the normal innominate vein or to properly lay the patch at its proximal end. The problem is not so much the actual length of the obstructed segment of vein, but that, if the segment has obviously extended into the innominate vein behind the manubrium of the sternum, the exposure needed to lay a patch appropriately or to connect proximal and distal normal vein is impossible to achieve. Therefore the regular incision needs to be extended into the sternum in order to expose the innominate vein, in some cases even up to the origin of the superior vena cava (Fig. 20.1a, b). The surgeon must keep in mind several caveats and injunctions when contemplating the use of this extension. First, once the sternum is entered, it is of the utmost importance in the postoperative period to keep the patient's arm immobilized for a minimum of 6 weeks postoperatively to allow the sternum to heal and to prevent a dehiscence. This will almost certainly occur if the patient is allowed to move the arm freely in all directions even if a proper sternal repair has been achieved at the end of the operation. Second, the extension should not be done until an attempt is made to use the regular incision to try to mobilize the vein into the operative field for placement of the venous patch (Fig. 19.11). Even when the clamps are already on the vein and the vein has been opened, extension of the incision can be carried out with the clamps in place until the manubrium of the sternum is divided. Because the patient has already been Heparinized, no thrombosis will occur.

Our technique for creating this extension has been previously described [1–4]. I prefer, first, to expose the sternal notch and to cut the ligaments at the top of the notch. Then, using blunt dissection (Fig. 20.2), a finger can be passed behind the manubrium of the sternum down towards the body of the bone connecting it with the dissection accomplished under the first rib stump laterally until the two ends of the dissection connect. At that point, I use a neuroairtome, because the surgeon can

J.E. Molina, *New Techniques for Thoracic Outlet Syndromes*,
DOI 10.1007/978-1-4614-5471-7_20,

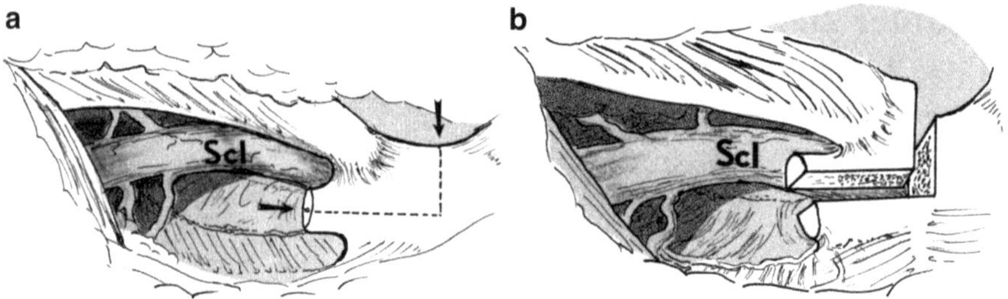

Fig. 20.1 Direction of the transmanubrium extension of the subclavicular incision. Scl = subclavian vein (**a** and **b**)

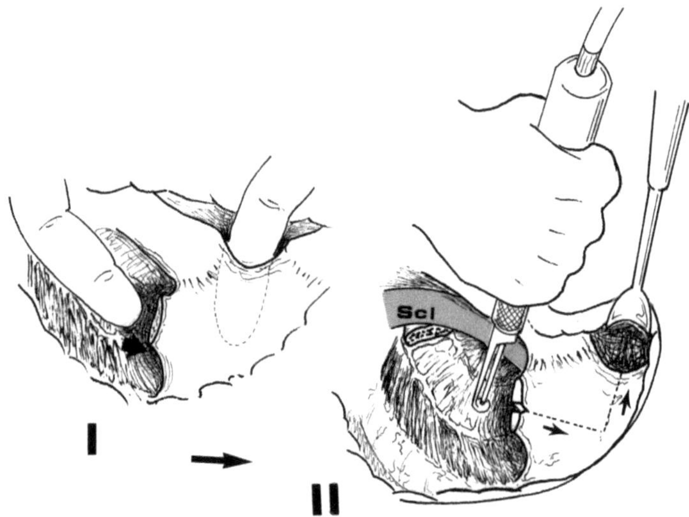

Fig. 20.2 Retrosternal blunt dissection behind the manubrium and under the stump of the first rib, followed by division of the sternum using the neuroairtome. Reprinted, with permission, from Molina JE. Approach to the confluence of the subclavian and internal jugular veins without claviculectomy. *Seminars in Vascular Surgery* 2000;13:10–19

turn it in a right angle direction without stopping the cutting mechanism. I start in the center of the rib stump and continue toward the middle of the sternum. Upon reaching it, I turn the neuroairtome at right angle and direct the cut towards the sternal notch. This is very easily done and doesn't cause complications. The bone is then divided using the cautery, and the retrosternal muscle as well as all connective tissue laying over the innominate vein is divided, also with the cautery.

A self retaining retractor is applied securing one side of the blades to the body of the sternum. The other blade goes to the separated wedge of the sternum manubrium thereby exposing the entire area (Fig. 20.3). The innominate vein is immediately visualized and dissected free of all connections. There is usually no need to ligate

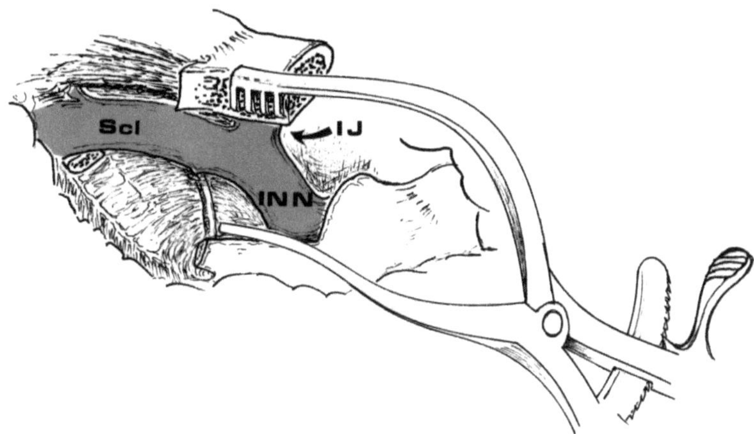

Fig. 20.3 After dividing the manubrium of the sternum a self-retaining retractor is placed with one blade on the body of the sternum and the other blade on the separated piece of the manubrium. The innominate and the subclavian veins are seen beneath readily accessible. Scl = subclavian vein, Ij = internal jugular vein, INN = innominate vein. Reprinted, with permission, from Molina JE. Approach to the confluence of the subclavian and internal jugular veins without claviculectomy. *Seminars in Vascular Surgery* 2000;13:10–19

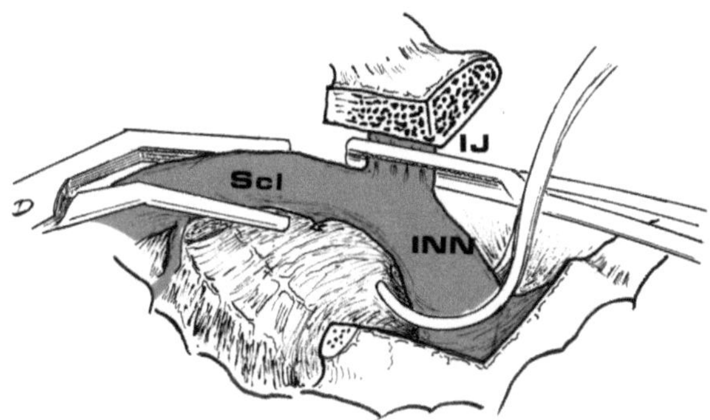

Fig. 20.4 Once the sternum is divided the veins are readily accessible to place clamps on the innominate as well as the subclavian and the internal jugular. Ij = internal jugular vein, Scl = subclavian vein, INN = innominate vein

any of the veins entering either the innominate vein or the subclavian. Occasionally, if the internal mammary vein may interfere with the exposure, it can be ligated, being careful to identify the phrenic nerve in order to prevent any damage to it. Once exposure is adequate, it is easy to move the clamp placed on the subclavian vein to a more medially position in a normal portion of the innominate vein (Fig. 20.4). The incision on the subclavian vein is now extended into the normal innominate vein, and then the saphenous vein patch is laid (Figs. 20.5, 20.6, 20.7, 20.8, 20.9, and 20.10).

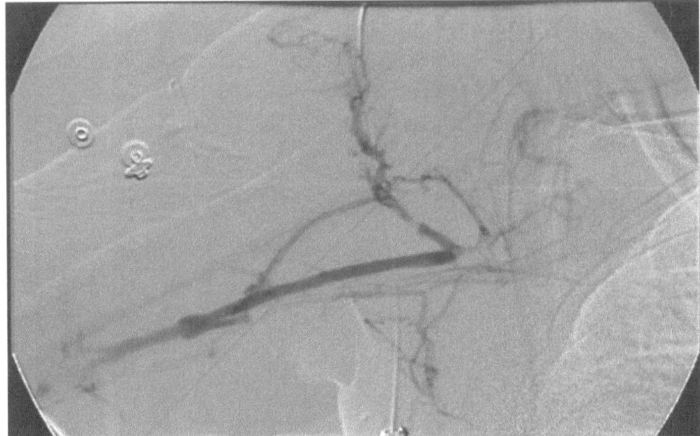

Fig. 20.5 A 22-year-old man with a very long segment of total obstruction of the right subclavian vein extending from the axillary to the innominate before implementing thrombolytic therapy. Reprinted, with permission, from Molina JE et al. Protocols for Paget–Schroetter Syndrome and late treatment of chronic subclavian vein obstruction. *Annals Thoracic Surgery* 2009;87;416–22

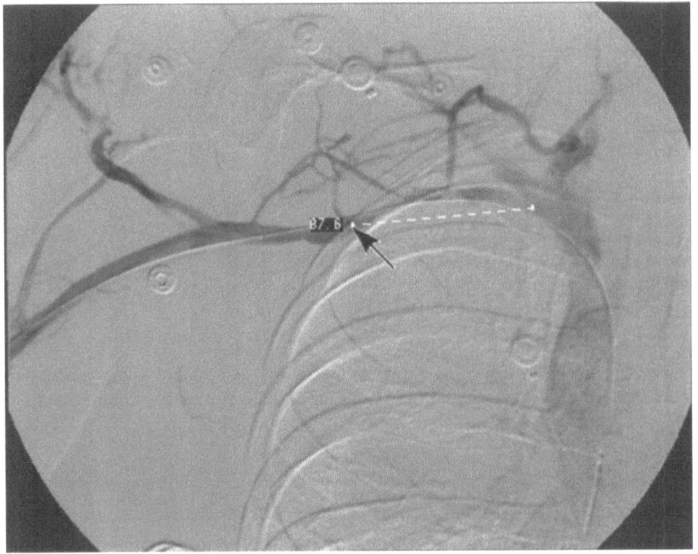

Fig. 20.6 After thrombolytic therapy measurement of the obstructed segment of the right subclavian vein reached 7.6 cm. Reprinted, with permission, from Molina JE et al. Protocols for Paget–Schroetter Syndrome and late treatment of chronic subclavian vein obstruction. *Annals Thoracic Surgery* 2009;87;416–22

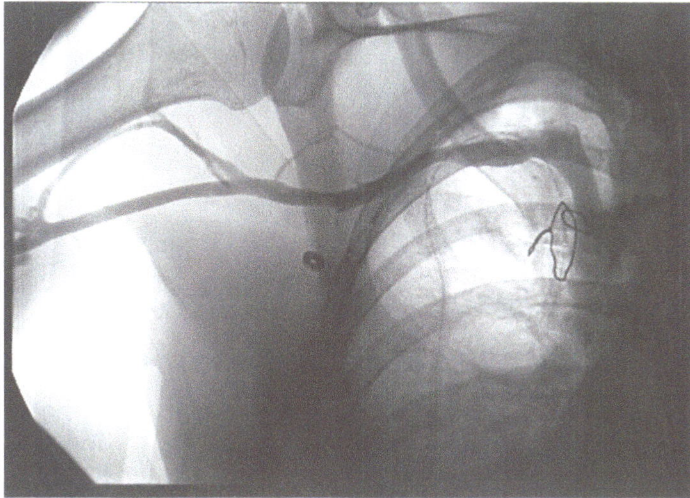

Fig. 20.7 Postoperative venogram of the same patient showing the reestablishment of the normal caliber of the subclavian vein reconnecting the axillary to the innominate. A transternal incision was used to approach the innominate vein and the two wires used for the reconstruction of the sternal incision are shown on the *right side* of the illustration

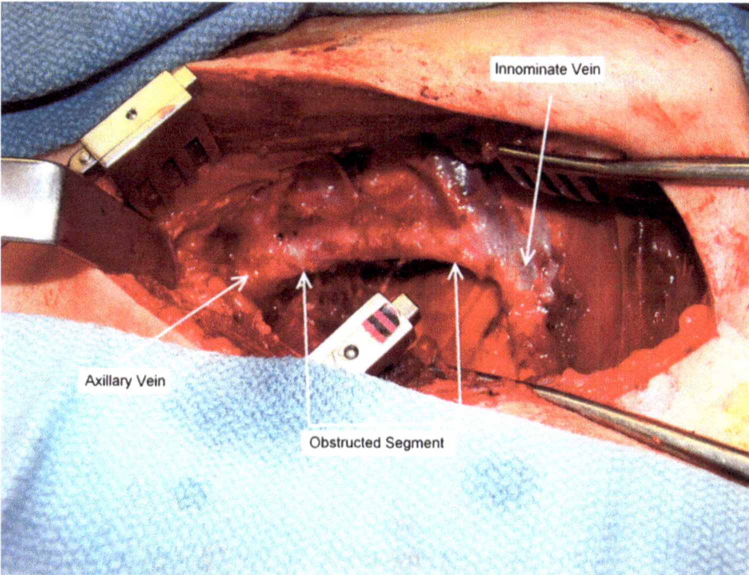

Fig. 20.8 Intraoperative photograph showing the obstructed vein segment

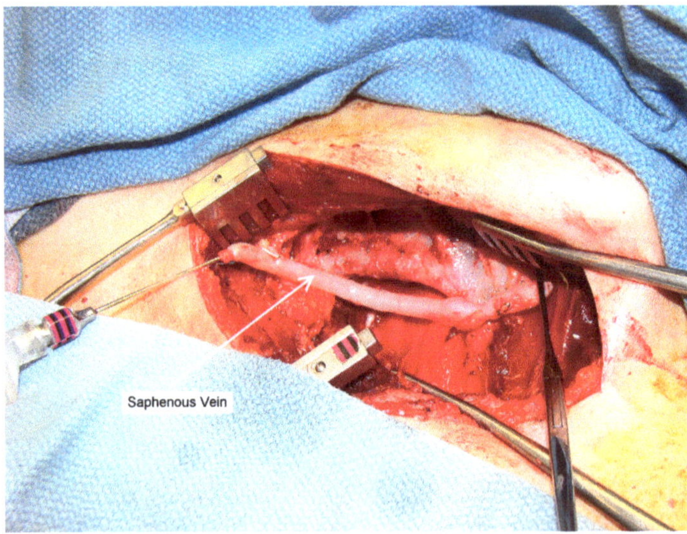

Fig. 20.9 The same patient showing the length of the saphenous vein graft needed to be used as a patch to enlarge the diameter of the subclavian reconnecting the axillary to the innominate vein

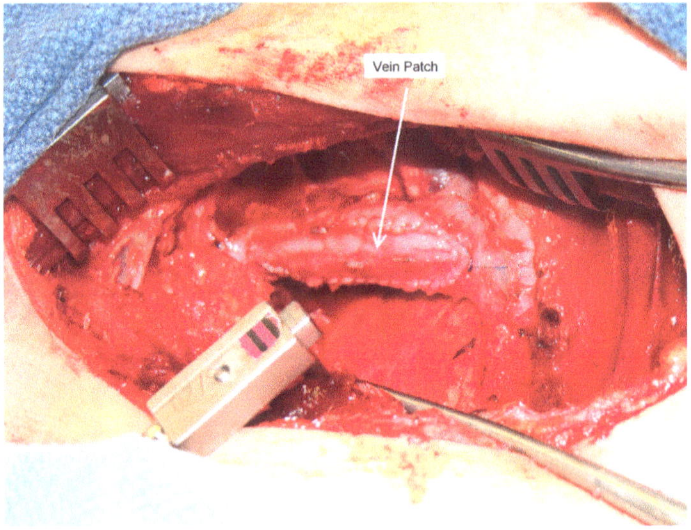

Fig. 20.10 Results after laying on the saphenous vein patch reconstructing the subclavian vein reestablishing its continuity. Reprinted, with permission, from Molina JE. Approach to the confluence of the subclavian and internal jugular veins without claviculectomy. *Seminars in Vascular Surgery* 2000;13:10–19

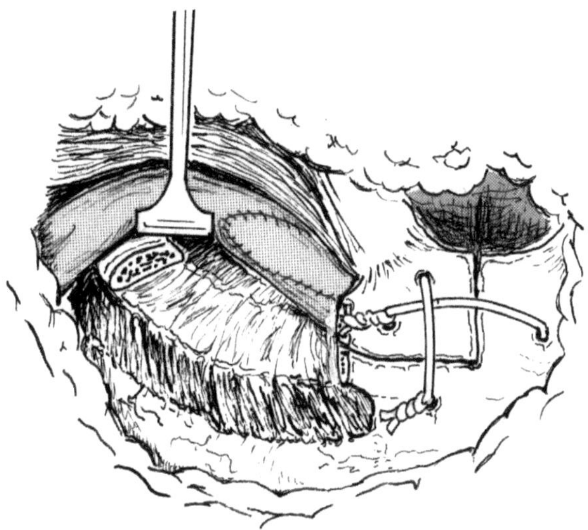

Fig. 20.11 The manubrium of the sternum has been already repaired and the fragments reapproximated. The subclavian vein can be seen behind with the inlaid patch to enlarge the diameter of the vein. The posterior stump of the first rib can be seen towards the *left side* of the illustration

In cases where metal stents have been previously implanted; they are cut along the vein past the end until normal innominate vein is entered.

Reconstruction of the sternal incision is accomplished using two wire stitches, one placed horizontally, and the other placed vertically (Fig. 20.11). The repair does require further dissection under the body of the sternum and under the half of the sternum opposite the separated segment. I prefer to place a malleable retractor underneath, the sternum and then to use a regular Yankee drill to create the appropriate holes through which the wire stitches are driven (see Fig. 20.12a–e). If the person is large, I use number 8 gauge stainless steel wire to do the reconstruction, but if the person is smaller, gauge number 6 is usually sufficient. After the closure of the sternum is completed, the rest of the incision is closed in the manner as already described. The surgeon should bury the twisted portion of the wire deeply under the muscle in order to prevent postoperative discomfort. This is particularly important if the patient is thin with only a layer of tissue over the sternum.

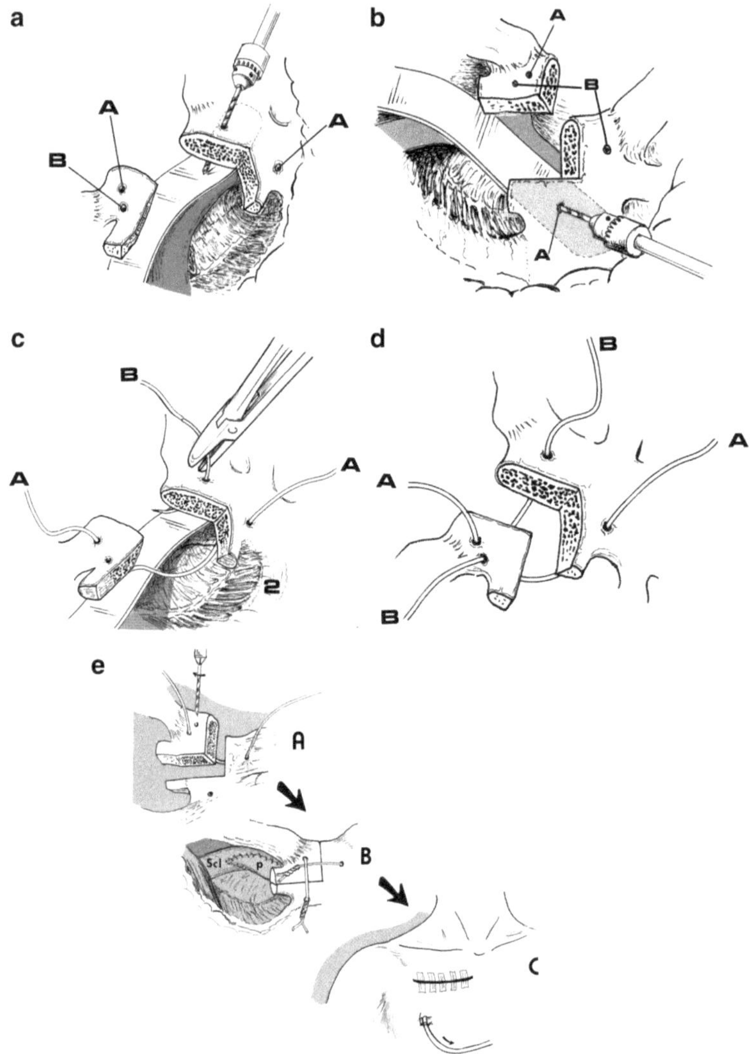

Fig. 20.12 (**a–e**) Sequential stages to repair the sternal incision protecting the mediastinal structures with malleable retractors. Using the Yankee drill holes are made in the manubrium as well as in the body of the sternum in order to place stainless steel wire sutures to reapproximate the two fragments of the sternum. Protecting the mediastinum with a malleable retractor. (B) The wire stitches are placed one horizontal and one vertical on the divided manubrium to reapproximate the fragments to their normal position. Reprinted, with permission, from Molina JE. Approach to the confluence of the subclavian and internal jugular veins without claviculectomy. *Seminars in Vascular Surgery* 2000;13:10–19 and Molina JE. Treatment of chronic obstruction of the axillary, subclavian and innominate veins. *International Journal of Angiology* 1999;8:87–90

References

1. Molina JE. A new surgical approach to the innominate and subclavian vein. J Vasc Surg. 1998;27:576–81.
2. Molina JE. Approach to the confluence of the subclavian and internal jugular veins without claviculectomy. Semin Vasc Surg. 2000;13:10–9.
3. Molina JE. Use of cryopreserved small aortic homografts for large vein replacement. Vasc Surg. 1999;33:545–55.
4. Molina JE. Operative technique of first rib resection via subclavicular approach. Vasc Surg. 1993;27:667–71.

Chapter 21
The Paraclavicular Approach

This approach is a combination of a supraclavicular and an infraclavicular incision. It is designed to expose the subclavian vein, the origin of the jugular vein and part of the innominate vein combined with a direct repair of the vein with or without patching, and to accomplish a thrombectomy combined with decompression of the thoracic inlet. The combination of these two incisions together allows for the simultaneous removal of the subclavius tendon, the costoclavicular ligament and the first rib. The approach was introduced by Cormier and Amrane [1] in order to achieve adequate exposure of the vessels of the thoracic outlet, used mostly for arterial repairs in patients with cervical ribs. The approach was later termed "Paraclavicular" by Thompson [2]. Satisfactory results have recently been reported by Melby [3]. The dual incision approach is adequate as long as the entire innominate vein does not need to be exposed, because it only provides limited visualization of the most proximal part of that vein. Therefore the approach is not sufficient in cases where the innominate vein has already endovascular stents placed or if the fibrous process has advanced into the innominate vein. A different incision must be utilized in these instances as described below. The paraclavicular approach has the merit of not dividing or partially removing the clavicle, which creates a very obvious chest deformity in the patient. The approach also allows the surgeon to repair directly the vein if necessary, and is preferable to any transaxillary approach to relieve the obstruction of the subclavian vein. Its clear limitations pertain to cases of chronic subclavian obstruction extending into the innominate (as noted above) or in patients who had been treated previously with implants and in whom there is a need to clamp the innominate vein near the superior vena cava in order to apply a patch to enlarge the vein. In such cases, we definitely prefer to use the transmanubrial extension of the subclavicular incision to obtain adequate control of the entire involved venous component.

J.E. Molina, *New Techniques for Thoracic Outlet Syndromes*,
DOI 10.1007/978-1-4614-5471-7_21,

References

1. Cormier JM, Amrane M, Ward A, Lavrian C, Gigou F. Arterial complications of the thoracic outlet syndrome: fifty-five operative cases. J Vasc Surg. 1989;9:778–87.
2. Thompson RW, Schneider PA, Nelken NA, et al. Circumferential venolysis and paraclavicular thoracic outlet decompression for "effort thrombosis" of the subclavian vein. J Vasc Surg. 1992;16:723–32.
3. Melby SJ, Vedantham S, Narra VR, Paletta GA, Khoo-Summers L, et al. Comprehensive surgical management of the competitive athlete with effort thrombosis of the subclavian vein (Paget-Schroetter syndrome). J Vasc Surg. 2008;47:809–21.

Chapter 22
The Transaxillary Approach

Many reports have been published using the transaxillary route to treat patients with Paget–Schroetter syndrome with various degrees of success. However, the objectivity of the results has been mostly based on symptomatic relief of those patients [1]. Some of the publications which have assessed the patency of the subclavian vein following this operation have shown a significant failure rate [2–6] (Fig. 22.1). We cannot recommend this type of approach based on those reports and also on our own experience seen patients weeks or even months after such intervention who have persisted showing signs of subclavian vein obstruction confirmed upon venography evaluation. The reason why this approach alone is not acceptable is because using the transaxillary route does not allow the surgeon to remove the subclavius muscle, the costoclavicular ligament nor the most anterior portion of the first rib at the sternal level (Fig. 22.2). These problems are seen more often in muscular individuals in which the retraction of the pectoralis major muscle is not sufficient to expose the cartilaginous portion of the first rib where the subclavius tendon and the costoclavicular ligament insert. Therefore often enough the surgeon after dividing the anterior scalene muscle resects the first rib but leaving part of the obstructive mechanism intact.

According to the illustration provided by Urschel in the Sabiston–Spencer textbook of surgery [7], to accomplish an effective removal of the first rib it is necessary to divide it anteriorly at the junction between the cartilaginous and osseous portions of the rib. However, this leaves behind a significant cartilaginous stump in continuity with the sternum, the site at which the tendon of the subclavius muscle and the costoclavicular ligament insert. Both constitute the vise mechanism compressing the vein against the rib remnant.

Our recommendation if the surgeon has used this transaxillary approach to relieve the subclavian vein extrinsic compression they must obtain an immediate postoperative venogram to assess whether the vein has been indeed decompressed and whether it has an acceptable caliber. If residual obstruction exists the patient

J.E. Molina, *New Techniques for Thoracic Outlet Syndromes*,

DOI 10.1007/978-1-4614-5471-7_22,

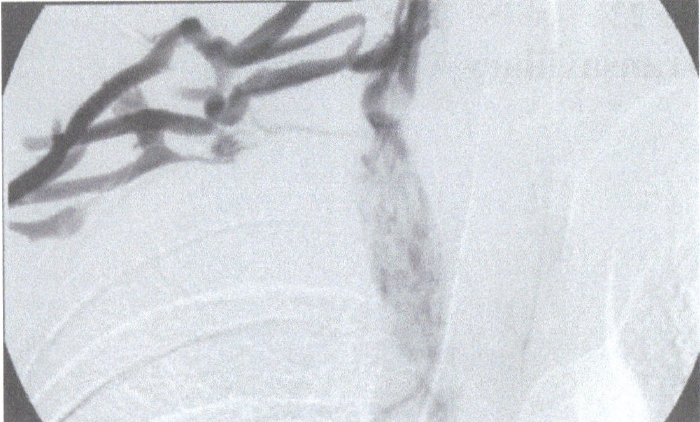

Fig. 22.1 A 33-year-old patient who suffered the original event 3 weeks earlier. After thrombolytic therapy, he underwent a transaxillary rib resection elsewhere. There is no identifiable axillary or subclavian vein, but only a network of collateral circulation making the case inoperable. There is faint visualization of the innominate vein extending into the superior venacava

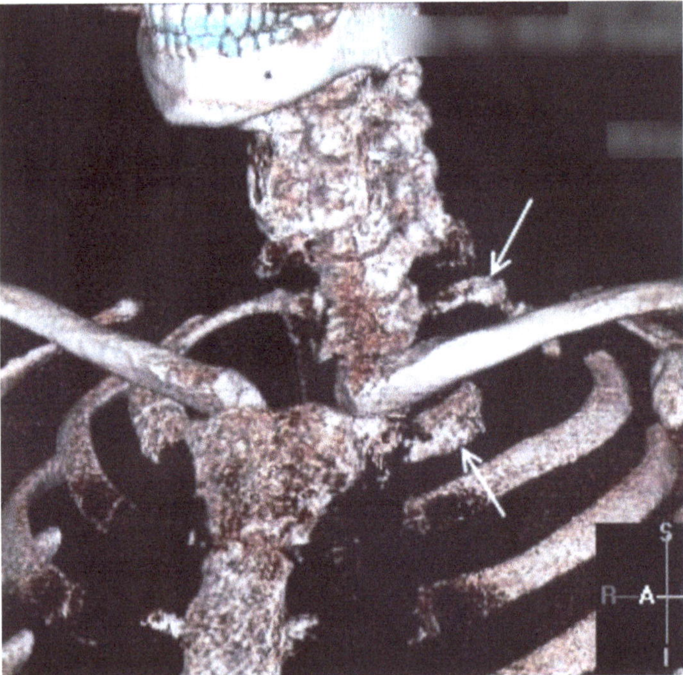

Fig. 22.2 A tridimensional CT scan of the chest shows the residual stumps of the first rib left after transaxillary resection (*arrows*). The anterior stump consists mainly of cartilage but this is the site where the subclavius tendon inserts as well as the costoclavicular ligament, and the cartilaginous portion constitutes the floor of the tunnel through which the subclavian vein is running. The posterior stump is mostly bone from an incomplete resection of the first rib. Reprinted, with permission, from Molina JE et al. Protocols for Paget–Schroetter Syndrome and late treatment of chronic subclavian vein obstruction. *Annals Thoracic Surgery* 2009;87:416–22

should be reoperated using an anterior subclavicular approach to remediate the problem instead of resourcing to balloon dilations or implant of stents that will not stay open due to the extrinsic compression that still remains [8]. The transaxillary approach is still used by many surgeons who had their surgical training in the last half of the past century and apply this decompressive operation designed to treat principally neurogenic arterial thoracic outlet syndromes extending its application to treat decompression of the subclavian vein which in our opinion is not adequate.

References

1. Urschel Jr HC, Razzuk MA. Paget-Schroetter syndrome: what is the best management? Ann Thorac Surg. 2000;69:1663–9.
2. DeLeon RA, Chang DC, Hassown H, Black JH, Roseborough GS, et al. Multiple treatment algorithms for successful outcomes in venous thoracic outlet syndromes. Surgery. 2009;145: 500–7.
3. Azakie A, McElhinney DB, Thompson RW, et al. Surgical management of subclavian-vein effort thrombosis as a result of thoracic outlet compression. J Vasc Surg. 1998;28:777–86.
4. Melby SJ, Vedantham S, Narra VR, Paletta GA, Khoo-Summers L, et al. Comprehensive surgical management of the competitive athlete with effort thrombosis of the subclavian vein (Paget-Schroetter syndrome). J Vasc Surg. 2008;47:809–21.
5. Machleder HI. Evaluations of a new treatment strategy for Paget-Schroetter syndrome: spontaneous thrombosis of the axillary-subclavian vein. J Vasc Surg. 1993;17:305–12.
6. Guzzo JL, Chang K, Demos J, Black JH, Freischlag JA. Preoperative thrombosis and venoplasty affords no benefit in patency following first rib resection and scalenectomy for subacute and chronic subclavian vein thrombosis. J Vasc Surg. 2010;52:658–63.
7. Urschel Jr HC, Razzuk MA. Ch. 18: Thoracic outlet syndrome. In: Sabiston DC, Spencer FC, editors. Surgery of the chest. 5th ed. Philadelphia: W. B. Saunders; 1990. p. 536–53.
8. Molina JE. Reoperations after failed transaxillary first rib resection to treat Paget-Schroetter syndrome patients. Ann Thorac Surg. 2011;91:1717–22.

Chapter 23
Reoperations After Failed Transaxillary First Rib Resection for Subclavian Vein Thrombosis

With increasing frequency we are seeing patients who have undergone a late transaxillary approach to decompress the subclavian vein several weeks after the patient has been initially diagnosed and treated with thrombolytic agents and the thrombus has resolved. This policy is wrong. This tendency occurs despite the current recommendation to operate on these patients immediately at the time of the original event even if the vein has been reopened using either thrombolytics or percutaneous thrombectomy catheter [1, 2]. The longer the waiting period for a definitive surgery, the lesser the chance of reestablishing a long-term patency and flow in the subclavian vein (Fig. 22.1). After the radiologist clears the vein, many of these patients are operated using the transaxillary route to remove the first rib on the thesis that simply by decompressing the thoracic inlet, the subclavian vein normal function will be reestablished. This is not the case. Because of the limitation of the transaxillary approach to reach the actual site of extrinsic compression of the vein caused by the subclavian tendon and the costoclavicular ligament, plus added incomplete removal of the anterior end of the rib, (Fig. 22.2) these patients often re-thrombose or remain obstructed shortly after the thrombolytic stage is completed [3]. When these patients return with the same symptoms they are frequently subjected to prolonged periods of anticoagulation hoping to have the vein re-canalize. It never occurs. Patients may also then be subjected to balloon dilation of the obstructed segment, often accompanied by the placement of endovascular stents [4–8]. Most commonly this does not resolve the problem: the site of the extrinsic compression has not been relieved, and therefore the stent kinks and the vein reobstructs again (Fig. 23.1). Some of the patients that we have seen have undergone multiple balloon dilations and stent placements in the same area with no success (Fig. 23.2). The patients are often left with no hope of having a cure for this disabling condition. We highly recommended that if this is the situation, the patient must be reoperated using a different approach namely the anterior route [3]. This is the only way to access the site of extrinsic compression with which the vein is still affected, because the ligaments are still intact and the cartilaginous most anterior portion of the first rib has not been removed. Often enough, the vein also needs to be repaired directly using a vein patch as described in Chap. 12. Afterward, if needed a stent can also be implanted.

J.E. Molina, *New Techniques for Thoracic Outlet Syndromes*,
DOI 10.1007/978-1-4614-5471-7_23, © Springer Science+Business Media New York 2013

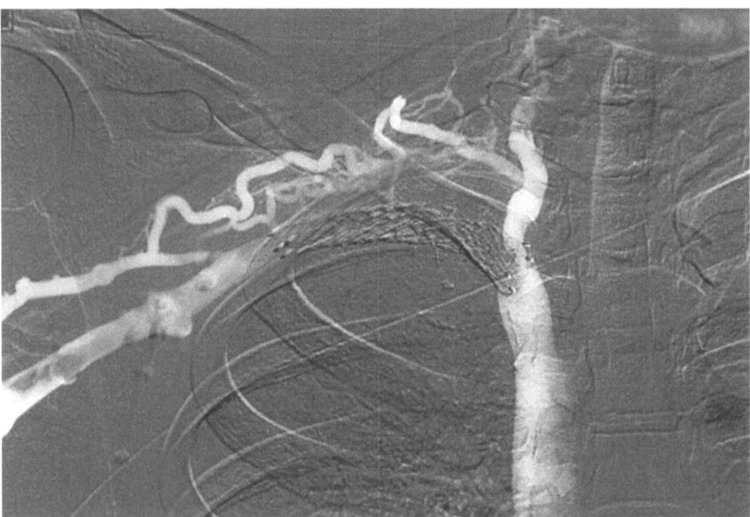

Fig. 23.1 Extensive recurrent thrombosis of a patient treated with only implant of stents without previously decompressing the thoracic inlet. The patient was still operable based on the patency of axillary vein

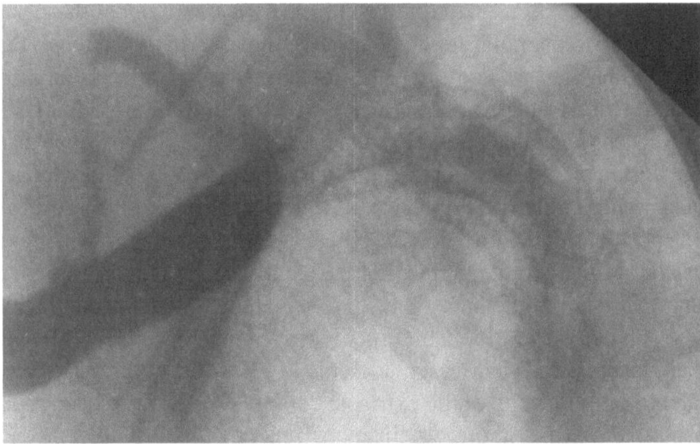

Fig. 23.2 A 49-year-old woman with total obstruction of the subclavian vein who had been previously treated with implants of three endovascular stents without decompressing the thoracic inlet anteriorly, but who still preserved the large caliber of the proximal axillary vein and therefore could still be reoperated reconnecting both ends of the vein. Reprinted, with permission, from Molina JE et al. Protocols for Paget–Schroetter Syndrome and late treatment of chronic subclavian vein obstruction. *Annals Thoracic Surgery* 2009;87;416–22

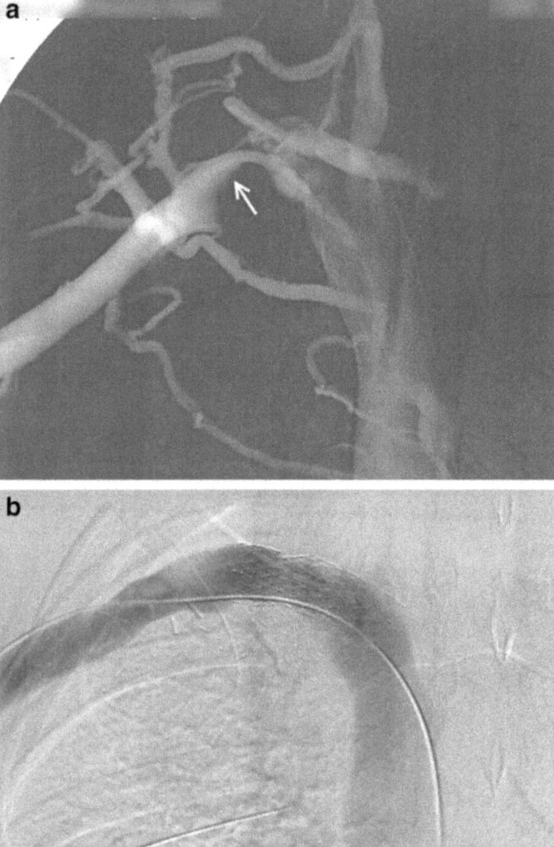

Fig. 23.3 (**a**) Venogram obtained after a transaxillary first rib resection for decompression of the subclavian vein. The indentation on the vein (*arrow*) is caused by the residual rib stump left anteriorly which continues to obstruct the vein significantly. (**b**) The same patient after reoperation undergoing anterior resection of the first rib, subclavius tendon, and costoclavicular ligament followed by implant of a vein patch and endovascular stent. The vein is perfectly open now

Some of these examples are shown in Figs. 23.3a, b and 23.4a, b. Figure 23.5 depicts some of the initial intraoperative findings showing the still persistent mechanical obstruction of the subclavian vein at the inlet. The results of reoperating these patients have been rewarding. However, not every patient is a candidate for this operation, particularly if the elapsed time between the initial thrombosis to the time of the transaxillary operation resection has been long. In a series of 16 patients seen with persistent obstruction of the subclavian vein after transaxillary resection of the first rib we were able to repair appropriately only 11 (Table 23.1). In five of them the vein was already extensively damaged and the fibrotic process had extended into the axillary vein with no adequate lumen was available to attempt any type of reconstruction. It is strongly suggested therefore that if the patient undergoes a

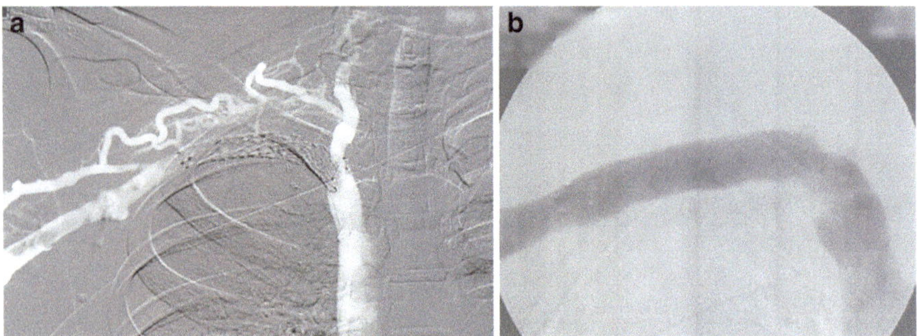

Fig. 23.4 (**a**) Status of the patient after transaxillary resection of the first rib leaving significant stump anteriorly. This was incorrectly treated with implants of two stents which predictably kinked and obstructed again. (**b**) Results after reoperating on this patient removing the anterior residual rib stump, placing a vein patch and implant of a stent, which at this time works very well since the extrinsic compression has been released. Reprinted, with permission, from Molina JE et al. Protocols for Paget–Schroetter Syndrome and late treatment of chronic subclavian vein obstruction. *Annals Thoracic Surgery* 2009;87;416–22

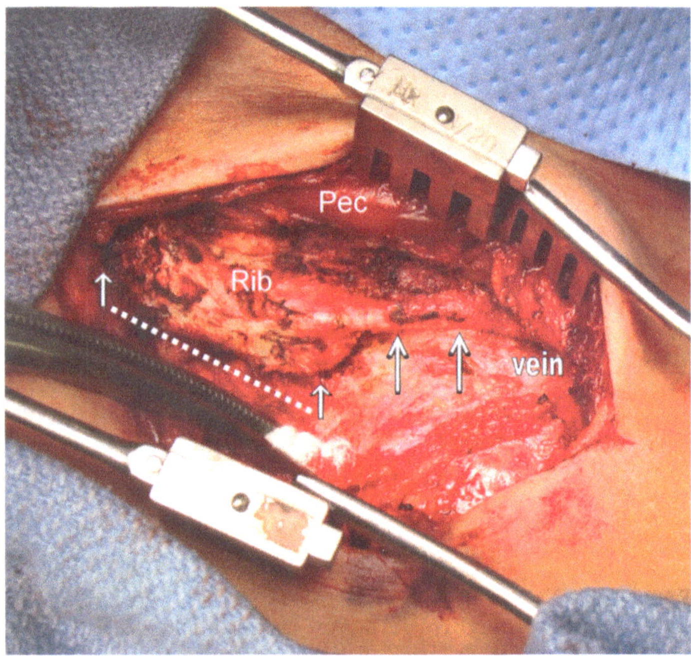

Fig. 23.5 An intraoperative photograph taken during a reoperation following a transaxillary resection of the rib which failed to decompress the subclavian vein. The anterior rib stump is quite significant shown by the *straight interrupted line* between the *arrows*. In addition the subclavius tendon is intact inserting on the rib stump (*longer arrows*) and the vein is still compressed under these structures. The pectoralis muscle (Pec) is shown above being retracted to expose the area. Reprinted, with permission, from Molina JE et al. Protocols for Paget–Schroetter Syndrome and late treatment of chronic subclavian vein obstruction. *Annals Thoracic Surgery* 2009;87;416–22

Table 23.1 Patients who underwent transaxillary first rib resection but were found to have occluded subclavian vein postoperatively, and were reoperated by us

Number	Age	Sex	Time of TARR after lytic therapy	Time found occluded	Number of repeated percutaneous manipulations	Stents implanted	Lapse before reoperation
1	26	F	5 weeks	Immediately	3	2	2 years 9 months
2	39	F	4 weeks	1 month	3	1	2 years 6 months
3	31	F	10 weeks	2 days	1	–	5 months
4	15	M	4 weeks	2 days	2	–	9 months
5	42	F	6 weeks	6 months	0	–	18 months
6	38	F	3 weeks	2 weeks	2	–	10 months
7	39	F	3 weeks	1 months	2	1	18 months
8	33	M	5 weeks	4 months	1	–	15 months
9	26	F	2 weeks	2 months	14	3	7 years
10	19	M	1 month	2 months	7	–	1 year
11	28	M	5 weeks	Immediately	6	–	9 months

TARR transaxillary rib resection

transaxillary resection of the first rib for Paget–Schroetter syndrome he/she should have an immediate postoperative venogram obtained to assess the status of the vein. If thrombosis persists, these patients should be reoperated using the anterior subclavicular route as soon as possible.

References

1. Machleder HI. Evaluations of a new treatment strategy for Paget-Schroetter syndrome: spontaneous thrombosis of the axillary-subclavian vein. J Vasc Surg. 1993;17:305–12.
2. Kunkel JM, Machleder HI. Treatement of Paget-Schroetter syndrome. A staged multidisciplinary approach. Arch Surg. 1989;124:1153–8.
3. Molina JE. Reoperations after failed transaxillary first rib resection to treat Paget-Schroetter syndrome patients. Ann Thorac Surg. 2011;91:1717–22.
4. Kreienberg PB, Chang BB, Darling RC, et al. Long-term results in patients treated with thrombolysis, thoracic inlet decompression, and subclavian vein stenting for Paget-Schroetter syndrome. J Vasc Surg. 2001;33((Suppl II)):100–5.
5. Urschel Jr HC, Patel AN. Paget-Schroetter syndrome therapy: failure of intravenous stents. Ann Thorac Surg. 2003;75:1693–6.
6. Hammer F, Becker D, Coffette P, et al. Crushed stents in benign left brachiocephalic vein stenosis. J Vasc Surg. 2000;32:392–6.
7. Bjarnason H, Hunter DW, Crain MR, et al. Collapse of a Palmaz stent in the subclavian vein. AJR Am J Roentgenol. 1993;160:1123–4.
8. Hall LD, Murray JD, Boswell GE. Venous stent placement as an adjunct to the staged, multimodal treatment of Paget-Schroetter syndrome. J Vasc Interv Radiol. 1995;6:565–70.

Chapter 24
Vein Replacement

In extreme cases [i.e., when the subclavian vein is totally obliterated (Fig. 24.1)] or when the vein segment has been repeatedly treated with multiple endovascular stents and has rethrombosed, it is impossible to operate and to lay a patch on the vein and expect it to function. In extreme cases in which the channel is practically nonexistent, but the inflow from the axillary vein measures at least 10 mm in diameter, it is feasible to remove the entire segment of the fibrotic vein and replace it with an interposition graft. At the present time there are no synthetic grafts that can function adequately in this position, so I have resorted to use of aortic homografts, usually descending thoracic aortic homografts harvested from cadavers of children [1–4]. They usually have a diameter of 10–12 mm roughly the size of the subclavian vein. It is also feasible to use an arterial homograft. Like iliac artery of adults, or even distal small abdominal aorta. The long term results of these homografts have initially been gratifying, however, within a year or 2, the walls of the homograft tend to become calcified and narrowed (Fig. 24.2a, b). If this occurs, it will be necessary to resort to endovascular stent placement in order to maintain a channel of proper caliber. So far this has been one solution to the problem. Fortunately, we have not had to use this approach often: in 25 years of experience treating total obstruction of the vein, we have only implanted 16 homografts (Fig. 24.3a–c). Our patency rates are 75% up to 7 years of follow-up. Patients treated in this manner should be followed on yearly intervals.

J.E. Molina, *New Techniques for Thoracic Outlet Syndromes*,
DOI 10.1007/978-1-4614-5471-7_24,

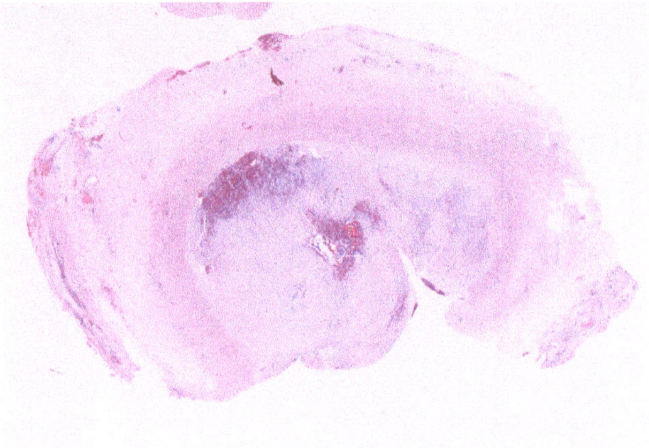

Fig. 24.1 Extensive fibrosis and organized thrombosis of the subclavian vein with no residual lumen. The vein was totally excised and the two ends of the still patent axillary vein and the innominate were reconnected using an arterial homograft

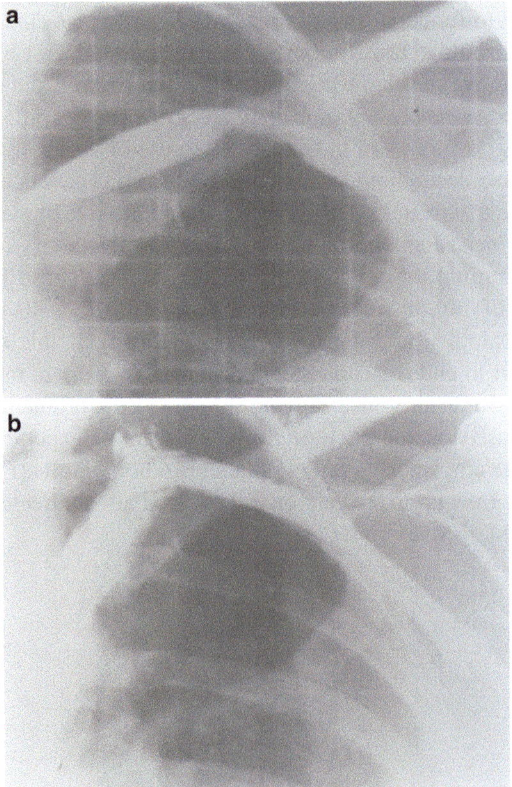

Fig. 24.2 (**a**) A stenosed aortic homograft in the left subclavian vein after 1 year of implant. (**b**) The same patient following balloon angioplasty and implant of an endovascular stent. Follow-up after 7 years stills shows good patency. Reprinted, with permission, from Molina JE et al. Protocols for Paget–Schroetter Syndrome and late treatment of chronic subclavian vein obstruction. *Annals Thoracic Surgery* 2009;87;416–22

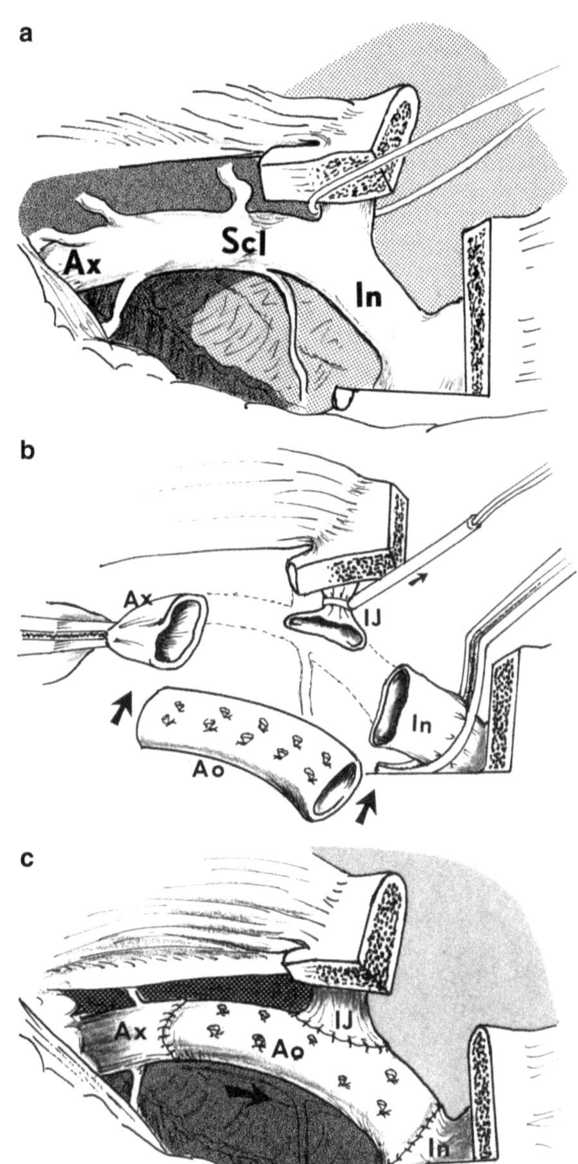

Fig. 24.3 (**a**) After implementing a transmanubrial division of the sternum and (**b**) retracting the upper section having the axillary and innominate veins cross clamped as well as the internal jugular vein isolated and occluded with a torniquette, a segment of a small segment of descending thoracic aorta homograft is being used to replace the subclavian vein that needed to be excised. Ax = axillary vein, Ij = internal jugular vein, In = innominate vein, Ao = aortic homograft. (**c**) Final reconstruction of the subclavian vein excision with reimplant of the internal jugular vein in an end to side fashion. Ax = axillary vein, Ao = aortic homograft, In = innominate vein. Reprinted, with permission, from Molina JE. Treatment of chronic obstruction of the axillary, subclavian and innominate veins. *International Journal of Angiology* 1999;8:87–90

References

1. Molina JE. A new surgical approach to the innominate and subclavian vein. J Vasc Surg. 1998;27:576–81.
2. Molina JE. Approach to the confluence of the subclavian and internal jugular veins without claviculectomy. Semin Vasc Surg. 2000;13:10–9.
3. Molina JE. Treatment of chronic obstruction of the axillary, subclavian, and innominate veins. Int J Angiol. 1999;8:87–90.
4. Molina JE. Use of cryopreserved small aortic homografts for large vein replacement. Vasc Surg. 1999;33:545–55.

Chapter 25
Postoperative Care: Anticoagulants, Pain Control, and Nursing Care

Anticoagulants

In the evening of the first postoperative day, the patient is started on anticoagulants, usually Coumadin at the dose of 10 mg unless the person has demonstrated previously sensitivity to the drug and may, therefore, need smaller amounts. At least 5 mg should be given orally that same evening. Also, the patient is started on oral Plavix (Clopidogrel), 75 mg daily. Lovenox is given subcutaneously at the dose of 40 mg bid for the first 48 h until the INR, which monitors the level of Coumadin reaches therapeutic levels (INR 2–3). The Dextran 40 which was started in surgery should also be continue at a rate of 15 cc per hour during the 48 h required for the Coumadin therapy to take effect [1]. No intravenous heparin is prescribed at any time and the patient is monitored with daily INR thereafter for the following 8–12 weeks (Table 25.1).

Chronic anticoagulation after surgery routinely should continue for 8 weeks. The use of stent implants requires a longer period (12 weeks) carried out using as noted, warfarin (Coumadin) to maintain an INR levels already specified.

With the advent of new anticoagulants that also have antiplatelet activity the postoperative anticoagulation of these patients is already changing. Among the Xa inhibitors like fondaparinux, rivaroxaban, and mainly dabigatran (Pradax) offer safer method of oral anticoagulation without the need for periodic blood test [2]. Those are already being used in preference to Coumadin and independent antiplatelet agents. Since the middle of 2011 therefore instead of Coumadin and Plavix we have started placing them on dabigatran at a dose of 150 mg orally twice a day. In several large randomized studies, Pradaxa has been proven to be more effective and safer than Coumadin when administered to patients with venous thrombosis or to prevent thromboembolism in patients with atrial fibrillation with no valvular procedures.

These new anticoagulants may be safer to use than warfarin. While we have not had any bleeding complications using warfarin for up to 12 weeks postoperatively, the risk is nevertheless still present. In addition the need to check INR levels weekly is both inconvenient for the patient and expensive.

J.E. Molina, *New Techniques for Thoracic Outlet Syndromes*,
DOI 10.1007/978-1-4614-5471-7_25,

Table 25.1 Anticoagulant therapy

	Dosage	
D. Postoperative (immediate)	Rheomacrodex 15 ml/h	
	Warfarin 10 mg Enoxaparin 30 mg Clopidogrel 75 mg	Same evening
E. Postoperative (early)	Rheomacrodex 15 ml/h for 48 h Warfarin daily to INR 2.0–3.0 Enoxaparin stopped at 48 h Clopidogrel 75 mg daily	
F. Postoperative (8 weeks)	Warfarin to INR 2.0–3.0 Clopidogrel 75 mg daily	

Pain Control

In the early post operative period the patient should remain on bed rest for the first 24 h at least during which time the patient is titrated using the PCA (Patient Control Analgesia) system to regulate the amount of pain medication needed. Routinely, we use Dilaudid because this opiate derivative is both effective and easy to manage. We prefer to maintain the PCA infusion for 48 h, at least. On the third day the patient is gradually switched to oral medication using a combination of Acetaminophen (Tylenol) with a narcotic, the most common of which are Percocet, Vicodin, Lortab, or Oxycodone. The patient is discharged home on one of these medications, which is then gradually tapered over the next 2 weeks.

Other

The Foley catheter which should be inserted at the time of surgery is left in place until the morning of the first postoperative day. The patient may ambulate but no exercise or physical therapy is needed the first few days after surgery. A post operative chest X-ray is taken routinely in the recovery room (Post Anesthesia Care Unit) to make sure no pneumothorax is present and that the lungs are properly expanded. The extrapleural drain (usually a round #19 Jackson-Pratt) is left in place until the total amount of drainage is less than 30 ml over a 24 h period. This usually occurs after 2 days, at which time the drain can be removed. If all goes well, however, at the end of the 3rd day the patient is discharged home on oral pain medications. The patient is then seen in the outpatient clinic for regular check ups at 2 weeks, and 8 weeks and, if necessary 12 weeks thereafter.

In cases operated for neurogenic-arterial thoracic outlet syndrome, the main issue is to control of pain for the reasons outlined above. The patient is advised to undertake only moderate activity for about 2 weeks and is cautioned not to drive a car for that same time period. In cases operated for subclavian vein thrombosis the two main points of concern are the pain control and maintenance of adequate anticoagulation levels using warfarin (Coumadin) at an INR between 2 and 3 for 8 weeks. However, if the patient underwent implant of an endovascular stent in the subclavian vein, in addition to a vein patch, then the recommended period of anticoagulation is extended to 12 weeks total. At the end of this time the anticoagulation regimen is discontinued completely.

In the unusual case in which the subclavicular incision was extended into the manubrium (as described above), the arm should be immobilized until the sternum is solidly healed. This usually requires 6 weeks using an arm sling which is kept in place at all times although it can be removed for certain minor activities (writing, typing, or eating). What patients must assiduously avoid however are all movements involving abduction of the arm away from the chest or over the head, which will place the sternal repair under extreme tension on and may lead to dehiscence of the incision. With this regimen, we have not had any problems of this nature and the sternum is usually solid at the end of 6 weeks. As far as wound care, the incisions are closed in the routine manner described in the operative technique section, and the skin is always sealed off using Dermabond. So therefore there are no skin stitches to be removed so that the status of its healing can be checked when the patient returns for routine appointments.

Postoperative physical therapy is usually not needed in cases involving subclavian vein obstruction. In some of the operations done for neurogenic-arterial thoracic outlet syndrome, however, physical therapy may be required for a period of about 6 weeks particularly if the patient has residual spasms of the muscles or needs help in restarting normal preoperative activity. At the end of 6 or 8 weeks, a routine chest X-ray is obtained to serve as a base line for future reference.

Follow-up duplex ultrasounds are obtained routinely on the patients undergoing surgery for subclavian vein obstruction, particularly if they underwent placement of an endovascular stent. The ultrasound done the day after any stent is implanted to verify patency of the vein, serves as a baseline for follow-up. A second ultrasound is obtained 4 weeks following the operation, the third ultrasound at the end of 8 weeks, and a fourth again at 12 weeks if the patient has been on anticoagulation therapy for that length of time. If, at the end of the 12 week period, the vein is patent and no signs of obstruction, the patient is considered cured. If doubts or questions persist, however, repeat ultrasounds can be obtained later. Usually however no ultrasounds are needed beyond 3 months.

References

1. Frost-Arner L, Bergquist D. Effects of heparin desmopressin, and isovolemic hemodihition with dextran on thrombus formation in synthetic vessel grafts inserted into the vena cava of the rabbit. J Vasc Surg. 1998;28:506–13.
2. Schulman S, Kearon C, Kakkar AK, et al. Dabigatran versus Warfarin in the treatment of acute venous thromboembolism. N Eng J Med. 2009;361:2342–52.

Part III
The Cervical Rib

Chapter 26
The Cervical Rib

A cervical rib is found in approximately 7% of patients suffering from thoracic outlet syndrome; [1–3] although its incidence has been previously reported as high as 25–33 % [4–7]. It is an extra rib that originates at the level of C7 and then extends laterally and anteriorly, fusing frequently with the anterior scalene muscle or inserting on top of the first rib behind the subclavian artery (Fig. 26.1). The rib is not always a bony structure readily visualized radiographically. Often enough, there is only a short bony structure resembling a horn on the X-ray arising from the C1 transverse process. Thereafter, however, it exists as a very strong ligament extending all the way down to the top of the first rib. Physiologically, it works exactly as a completely ossified structure would. In 1869, Gruber proposed a classification of cervical ribs [8, 9] based on the amount of bone present and on the thickness of the rib like structure. (Fig. 26.2) The virtue of this classification it that it shows that, even when the radiographic exam only demonstrates prominence of the C7 transverse process, most often a strong fibrous ligament does actually extend from the tip of that process all the way to the top of the first rib, none of which can be visualized on the plain X-ray exam (Fig. 26.3).

According to Adson and Coffey [10], Coote was the first to report resecting a cervical rib (1861). He used the supraclavicular route as his approach to its removal [11]. At the beginning of the twentieth century surgeons uniformly utilized the transverse incision above the clavicle, later modified as an "L" shaped extending it along the trapezius ridge [12]. Because the mechanism of compression of the brachial plexus was fairly well understood at that time, the first rib was then removed from the anterior tubercle (where the anterior scalene muscle inserts) towards its posterior end at the junction with the transverse process of the vertebral body. One of the most specific descriptions of how to remove this portion of the rib was made by Stiles in a textbook by Jones and Lovett [13]. Many text books of surgery also indicated that this approach could relieve the compression of the brachial plexus. For all of these reasons this approach represented the gold standard of treatment well into the twentieth century.

J.E. Molina, *New Techniques for Thoracic Outlet Syndromes*,

DOI 10.1007/978-1-4614-5471-7_26,

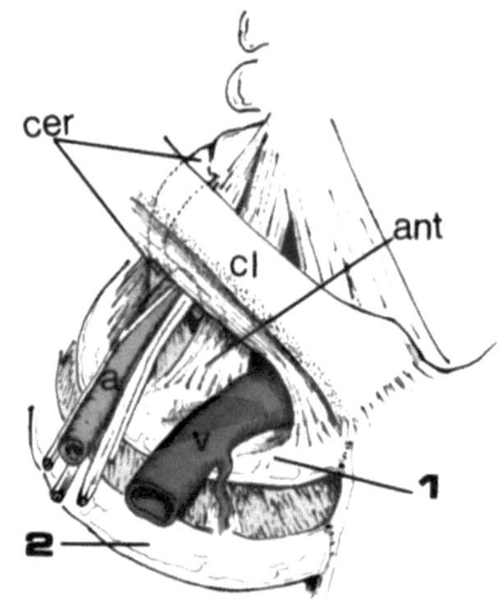

Fig. 26.1 The thoracic outlet in the presence of cervical rib (cer) Cl = clavicle, ant = anterior scalene muscle. Reprinted, with permission, from Molina JE et al. Protocols for Paget–Schroetter Syndrome and late treatment of chronic subclavian vein obstruction. *Annals Thoracic Surgery* 2009;87;416–22

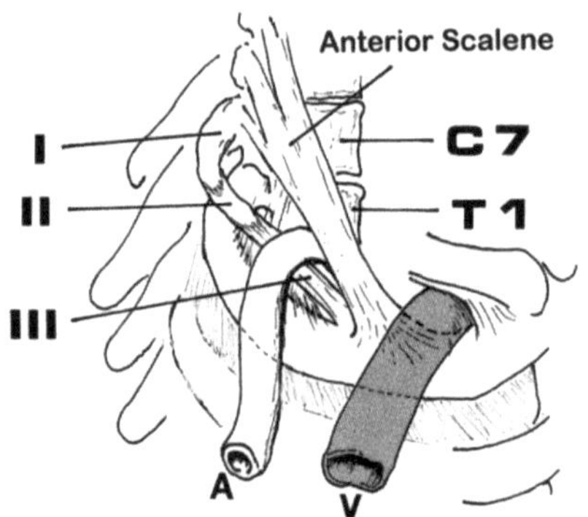

Fig. 26.2 Illustration depicting the degrees (I, II, and III) of cervical rib development according to the Grubber classification (see text). C7 = 7th cervical vertebral body, T1 = 1st thoracic vertebral body. A = subclavian artery, V = subclavian vein

One of its drawbacks, however, is the obviously visible scar left on the anterior neck. Women (who constitute the majority of the afflicted patients) objected in particular to the disfigurement, which is especially prominent if an “L” shaped incision has been used. Roos and Saunders [14, 15] therefore proposed to address the problem by using a transaxillary approach to first rib removal for whatever reason (compression along or compression from a cervical rib). Unfortunately, experience has shown that removing a cervical rib via the transaxillary approach can be even more difficult than using it to remove the first rib (which is in a lower location). Attempting to expose it all the way up to its origin may prove anatomically impossible in many instances. We believe that the supraclavicular operation is preferable over the transaxillary route for neurogenic thoracic outlet syndrome because it allows the surgeon to access both the cervical and the first ribs. However, our combined approach of transaxillary and posterior limited transverse incision, as described in the section of neurogenic thoracic outlet syndrome, has the advantage of being

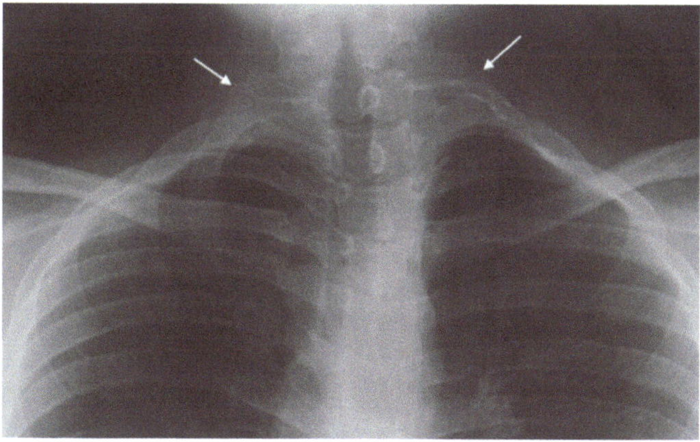

Fig. 26.3 Bilateral cervical ribs. Although the right rib is complete, the patient was symptomatic only on the left side

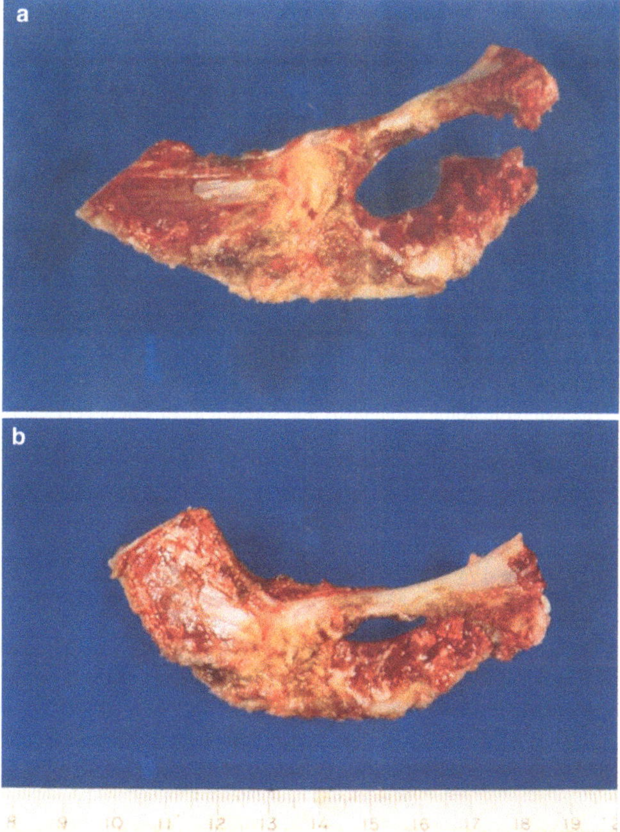

Fig. 26.4 (**a**) Anterior view of a surgical specimen showing the cervical rib inserting on the superior aspect of the first rib, in the tubercle where the anterior scalene muscle inserts as well. This constitutes a type 3 Grubber classification of cervical rib. To the left of the illustration is the sternal insertion of the first rib and to the right the insertion of both ribs on the vertebral column. (**b**) Inner aspect of the same specimen showing the fan extension of the insertion fibers of the anterior scalene muscle

cosmetically acceptable and allowing complete removal of the cervical rib along with the first thoracic without risking any neurologic or vascular injuries [16] (Fig. 26.4). Excellent descriptions of the cervical rib anatomy and pathology can be found in the publications of Murphy [17], Naffziger and Grant [18], and Thorburn [19].

References

1. Roos DB. The place for scalenectomy and first-rib resection in thoracic outlet syndrome. Surgery. 1982;92:1077–85.
2. William HT, Carpenter NH. Surgical treatment of the thoracic outlet compression syndrome. Arch Surg. 1978;113:850–2.
3. Molina JE. Personal records 1987–2012 (unpublished)
4. Urschel Jr HC, Paulson DL, McNamara JJ. Thoracic outlet syndrome. Ann Thorac Surg. 1968;6:1–10.
5. Green RM, McNamara J, Ouriel K. Long-term follow-up after thoracic outlet decompression: an analysis of factors determining outcome. J Vasc Surg. 1991;14:739–46.
6. Reilly LM, Stoney RJ. Supraclavicular approach for thoracic outlet decompression. J Vasc Surg. 1988;8:329–34.
7. Bertelsen S. Neurovascular compression syndromes of the neck and shoulder. Acta Chir Scand. 1969;135:137–48.
8. Gruber W. Über die Halsrippen des Menschen Mem l'Acad Imperial des Sci. St. Petersburg; 1869, vol 7:series 13 No 2.
9. Gruber W. Vortäuschung einer Fractur der ersten Rippe durch eine kurze supernumeräre Rippe. Arch Pathol Anat Physiol Klin Med. 1865;32:108.
10. Adson AW, Coffey JR. Cervical rib. A method of anterior approach for relief of symptoms by division of the scalenus anticus. Ann Surg. 1927;85:839–57.
11. Coote H. Pressure on the axillary vessels and nerves by an exostosis from a cervical rib interference with the circulation of the arm. Removal of the rib and exostosis. Recovery. Med Times Gaz. 1861;2:108.
12. Keen WW. The symptomatology, diagnosis and surgical treatment of cervical ribs. Am J Med Sci. 1907;133(2):173–218.
13. Jones R, Lovett RW. Orthopedic surgery. New York: Wm Wood & Co; 1923. p. 549–51.
14. Roos DB. Transaxillary approach for first rib resection to relieve thoracic outlet syndrome. Ann Surg. 1966;163:354–8.
15. Sander RJ, Pearse WH. The treatment of thoracic outlet syndrome: a comparison of different operations. J Vasc Surg. 1989;10:626–34.
16. Molina JE. Combined posterior and transaxillary approach for neurogenic thoracic outlet syndrome. J Am Coll Surg. 1998;187:39–45.
17. Murphy JB. The clinical significance of cervical ribs. Surg Gynecol Obstet. 1906;3:514–20.
18. Naffziger HC, Grant WT. Neuritis of the brachial plexus mechanical in origin: the scalenus syndrome. Surg Gynecol Obstet. 1938;67:722–30.
19. Thorburn W. The seventh cervical rib and its effects upon the brachial plexus. Med Chir Tran. 1905;88:109–25.

Chapter 27
Fusion of Ribs

One of the most frequent congenital anomalies seen in this anatomic area is a fusion of the first and second ribs. This may occur throughout the entire length of the rib or only in a segment (Fig. 27.1). Patients with this anomaly usually become symptomatic in early youth, especially when they become involved in sports and other recreational physical activities.

The most usual course is to become very symptomatic at an early age. The youngest we have seen occurred at 12 years, but symptoms can develop at almost any time. The diagnosis is easily made with X-ray studies particularly using tridimensional reconstruction of a CT scan. When the fusion of the two ribs occurs for a short distance in the mid portion of each, the fusion can be divided surgically sparing the second rib and removing only the first. However, if the fusion is complete from back to front (Fig. 27.2). the ribs are frequently not only fused, but also twisted over each other. In such cases, both ribs need to be removed. Technically it is advisable to use our dual transaxillary and posterior incision behind the trapezius ridge. During the transaxillary stage, it is safer to start by dissecting the inferior border of the second rib to create an extrapleural space. Dissection is then advanced superiorly to involve the first rib as well. As the anterior surface of the fused rib is approached, the vein can be retracted superiorly. It must be noted, however, that the anterior scalene muscle is often ossified as well, and must be divided either with a rongeur or rib cutter. Once the rib is divided anteriorly, the posterior incision is carried out in the usual fashion and the first and the second ribs are dissected free and removed en block (Figs. 27.2 and 27.3). Outcomes are usually very satisfactory the patients experience symptomatic relief almost immediately. It is preferable to operate on these cases when the diagnosis is made because, as the patients grow older the ribs widen and it is very difficult to find the proper instruments to divide them. It is also more difficult to protect the vascular structures in the apex of the chest under these conditions.

J.E. Molina, *New Techniques for Thoracic Outlet Syndromes*,
DOI 10.1007/978-1-4614-5471-7_27,

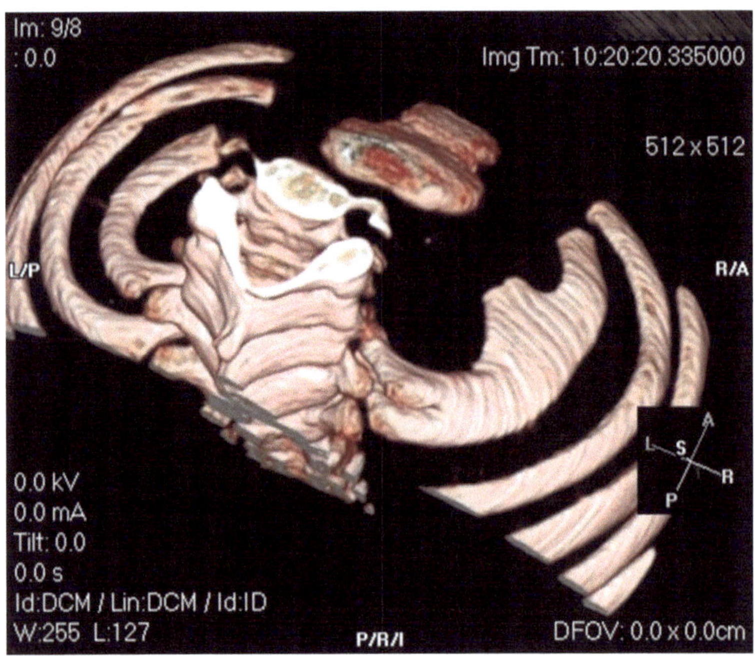

Fig. 27.1 Right-sided fusion of first and second ribs in a 12-year-old child

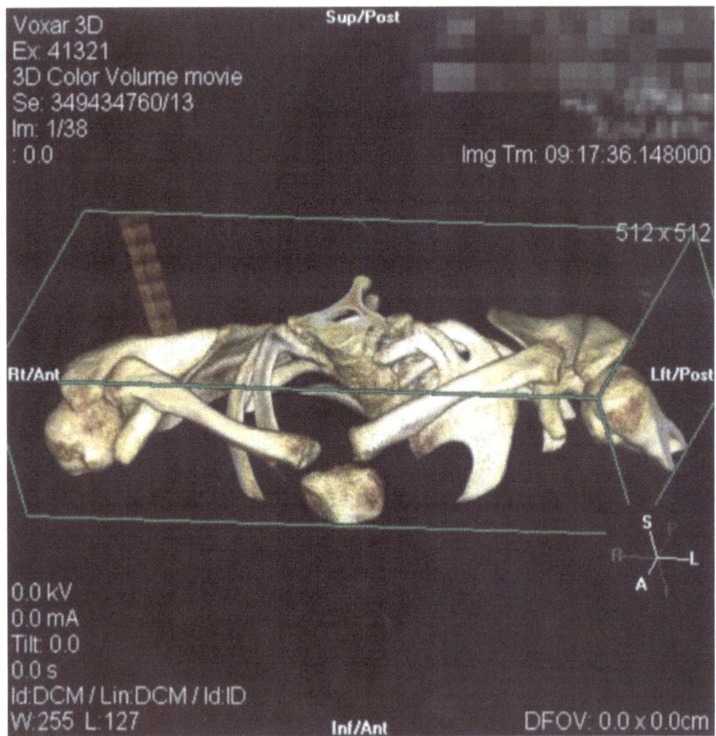

Fig. 27.2 Left-sided fusion of first and second ribs in a man who became symptomatic until he began physical demanding work. His symptoms were completely relieved after removal of the fused ribs

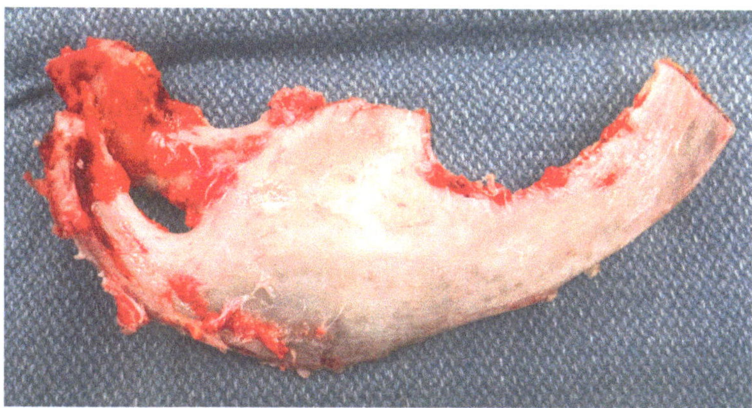

Fig. 27.3 Removed specimen. The vertebral insertions of the ribs appear on the left side and the sternal single insertion to the sternum on the right side

Index

J.E. Molina, *New Techniques for Thoracic Outlet Syndromes*,
DOI 10.1007/978-1-4614-5471-7, © Springer Science+Business Media New York 2013

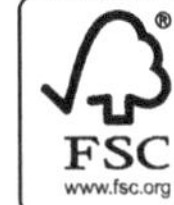

MIX
Papier aus verantwortungsvollen Quellen
Paper from responsible sources
FSC® C105338

If you have any concerns about our products,
you can contact us on
ProductSafety@springernature.com

In case Publisher is established outside the EU,
the EU authorized representative is:
Springer Nature Customer Service Center GmbH
Europaplatz 3, 69115 Heidelberg, Germany

Printed by Libri Plureos GmbH
in Hamburg, Germany